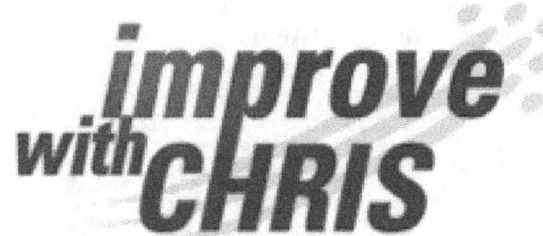

Client PROgression Journal

Powered by

PROformance
Training
Systems

Client's Name_____

Email_____

Phone_____

PROformance Training Systems				
Mechanical	**Learn**	**Prepare**	**Fortify**	**Potential**
	Mobility Sets 2-3 Reps 12-15 Rest 60s Inten. 1-40%	*Functional Stability* Sets 3 Reps 12-15 Rest 30-45s Inten. 50-75%	*Muscular Endurance* Sets 3 Reps 12-15 Rest <30s Inten. 50-75%	*Max Power* Sets 3-6 Reps 1-10 Rest 3-5min. Inten. 45% or 10% BW
	Corrective Sets 2-3 Reps 12-15 Rest 60s Inten. 40-60%	*Neuromuscular Efficiency* Sets 3 Reps 12-15 Rest 30-45s Inten. 50-75%	*Hypertrophy* Sets 3-4 Reps 4-12 Rest 45s-2.5min. Inten.75-85%	*Advanced Movement Systems* Sets 3-6 Reps 1-10 Rest 3-5min. Inten. 100%
			Heavy Power Sets 4-6 Reps 1-4 Rest 3-5min. Inten.85-100%	
Metabolic	**Learn**	**Prepare**	**Fortify**	**Potential**
	Metabolic Stimulation HR 50-60% Reps = Varies Rest Ratio = Rest as needed	*Aerobic Elevation* HR 60-80% Reps 1 Rest Ratio = Steady State	*Threshold Development* HR 80-92% Rest Ratio 5:1	*Specific Movements* As appropiate
			Aerobic Capacity HR 92-98% Rest Rat. 2:1-1:1	*Specific Skills* As Appropriate
			Anaerobic Expansion HR 95-100% Rest Rat. 1:3-1:5	
ATP Replenishment	**Muscle Fiber Activity**			
50% = 20-30s 75% = 40s 85-90% = 60s 100% = 3min.	Type I | Activation = 0%, Peak = 60%, Max = 80% Type IIa | Activation = 60%, Peak = 85%, Max = 95% Type IIb | Activation = 90%, Peak = 100+, Max = 100+			

PROformance Training Systems

Based on years of training experience as well as a vast knowledge of sports & exercise science, I have developed PROformance Training Systems. PROformance Training Systems is my results proven method for progressing all of my athletes. The system follows a sound set of principles that allow me to progress my athletes safely and effectively through "Themes." Each theme has a specific goal and rules that must be followed to obtain that goal. Athletes must master one theme before progressing up the "PROgression Model." By mastering each theme in their specific order, it ensures higher athletic success with reduced chance of injury. PROformance Training Systems™ also has a set of checks and balances to ensure athletes are not back tracking or steering off course. PROformance Training Systems™ is the system that this journal is based on. The following flowcharts explain the logic behind the method. A sound understanding of the flowcharts is necessary before going into the PROformance Training Systems™ Progression Model itself.

PROformance Foundations Flowchart I

When it comes to improving ourselves as athletes, the appropriate steps should be taken in the correct Sequence. These steps are functional movement, mechanical integrity, metabolic capacity, and specific skill in that order. Functional movement is the ability to move the body through basic practical movement patterns properly without pain. This step should not be viewed as exercise but rather as learning. If we want to advance towards athletic excellence, we must first learn the proper functional movements and be able to complete them free of pain. The second step is mechanical integrity. Once correct movement patterns are put in place, the mechanical structures of the body (muscles, tendon, ligaments, and fascia) must be fortified. Heavy and intense resistance training should not be performed without first establishing mechanical integrity. Moreover, it would not make sense to progress someone towards cardiovascular fitness if their body is not ready to handle the stress of the associated workload. Therefore, adequate time must be taken to ensure appropriate mechanical integrity prior to implementing the repetitive movements and high volume loads associated with cardiovascular training. Next, metabolic capacity can be established. The metabolic pathways can be anaerobic or aerobic in nature, they are the phosphagen system (anaerobic), glycolysis (anaerobic), or aerobic system (aerobic). Proper metabolic pathways should be trained for particular sports and goals. Olympic lifting energy pathways are very different from distance running. Therefore they should be handled differently, however each discipline should be developed with equal importance.

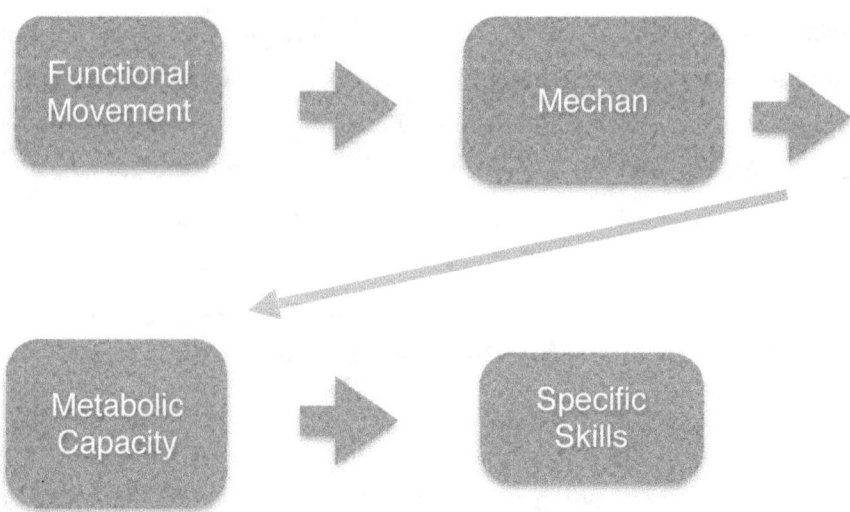

Finally, specific skills can be obtained. To truly master and excel in a specific skill of sport and athleticism, one must first acquire the ample functional movement, structural integrity, and metabolic capacity associated with that skill. Always re-assessing the steps to make certain one does not develop a weakness in one area by focusing too strongly on another. Skipping any one of these steps will only set you up for injury or sub-optimal performance. For optimal athleticism to be achieved, the proper sequence of athletic progression must be followed. Just as you cannot win a war without an army, can't have an army without soldiers, and can't have soldiers without proper training and tools. The body cannot reach its athletic potential without first attaining specific skills, it can't reach the skills without the metabolic capacity to perform, it can't perform without the structural integrity to hold it all together and allow it to move, and can't move correctly and efficiently if it does not have proper movement patterns and stability. Follow the proper progression and ensure optimal performance.

PROformance Foundations Flowchart II

Control & Capacity

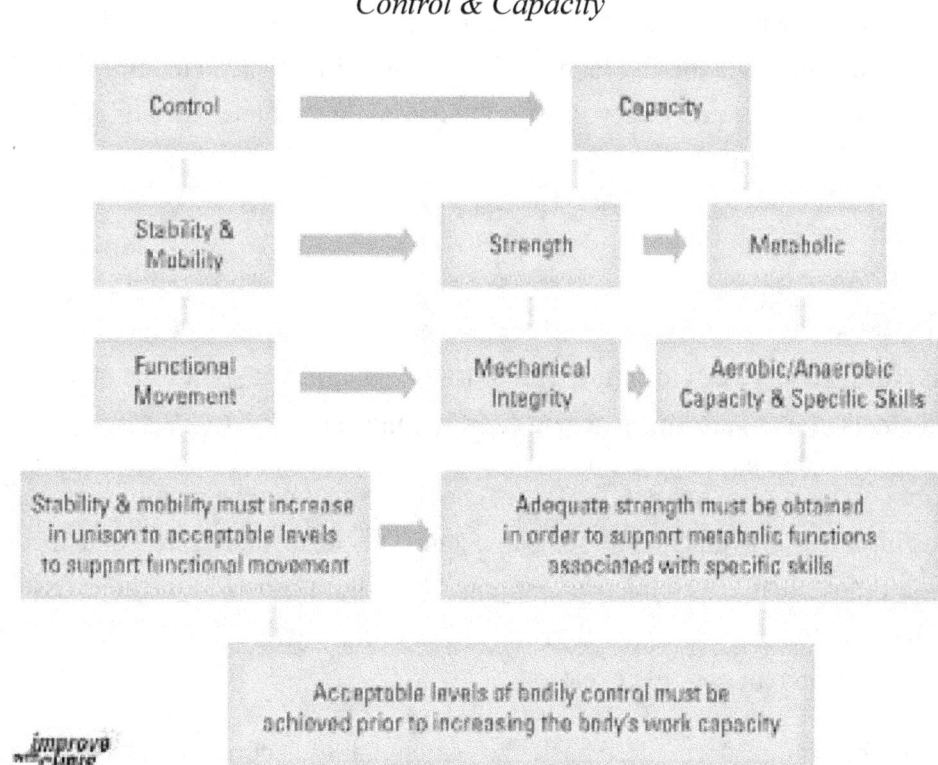

Excellence is reaching the pinnacle of a discipline and mastering all the steps along the way. Achieving excellence in human performance is built on solid foundations. The roots of these foundations are control and capacity. Control is the body's ability to adequately manage itself through sufficiently and simultaneously limiting and allowing motion. Capacity on the other hand is the ability to elevate the body to heightened levels of control. Efficient control must be obtained prior to increasing capacity in order to support the repetitive nature of metabolic functions associated with specific skill development while avoiding injury due to muscle imbalances and poor Arthrokinematics (joint movement) that can be amplified during repetitive movements (i.e., high volume training). The basis of control is stability and mobility. Stability is the product of proprioception (the body's self- awareness in space) and timing (properly adjusting the body within space as a result of proprioceptive feedback). When proprioception and stability are working together in harmony, the body is able to achieve controlled functional movement. Mobility is the second half of control's source. Mobility is simply the freedom to move without restrictions. Sufficient mobility is mandatory to achieve the greatest amount of control possible. Stability & mobility must increase in unison. As you achieve new levels of mobility, you must be able to stabilize the range of motion; and as you improve stability, it allows you to support greater mobility. Remember, quality before quantity (Cook, 2010). Once ample control is attained, the athlete can start enhancing their capacity. Capacity is the product of strength and metabolic capability. Strength is the aptitude to effectively execute stability and mobility at elevated levels and must be obtained prior to increasing metabolic ability in order to ensure proper movement as fatigue settles in and thus avoid injury. Metabolic, is the ability to sustain feats of strength over a sustained period of time. It is during metabolic amplification that the athlete reaches their potential. However, that potential cannot be reached or sustained without first adequately building the prior steps (stability, mobility, and strength). Metabolic function can be either aerobic or anaerobic depending on the demands of the sport, which leads to specific skills development. The training system being utilized should be sport specific the whole way through. When functional movement, mechanical integrity, and capacity are finally achieved, the athlete can begin fine tuning their sport specific skills. This is the time to train the specific demands of the physical feat(s) associated with your sport and when the athlete can achieve their true peak performance.

PROformance Foundations Flowchart III

How Our Basic Survival Instincts Lead to Injury The following diagram displays the chain of events that allow our basic survival instincts to instigate injury during exercise and sport.

Humans by nature are creatures of extreme efficiency. As a result we take the path of least resistance. If we are weak in certain areas improper movement patterns can occur. This leads to muscle imbalances and poor Arthrokinematics (joint movement), which leads to injury. Our natural survival instincts tell us to avoid movements that cause pain or are unfamiliar even if they are natural (the way it is "supposed" to be). This leads to further pain and injury; creating an ongoing cycle.

We must re-educate our body to perform these basic movement patterns correctly in order to reduce injury and maximize performance. By relearning proper biomechanics from the beginning we are allowing our body to perform in harmony.

Survival Mechanism

PROformance Training Systems™ is designed to do just that, re-balance our body, strengthen its parts, and fine tune it towards athletic success.

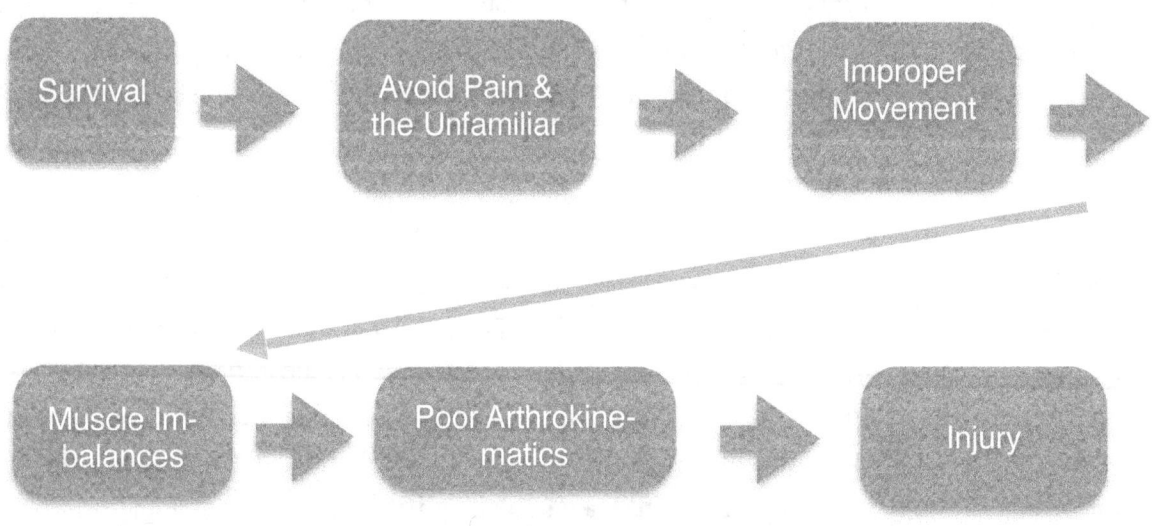

The PROformance Training Systems PROgression Model

PROformance Training Systems

Functional Integrated Movements	Mechanical	Theme	Metabolic	Constant Evaluation & Systems Adaption
	Advanced Movement Systems & Max Power	Potential	**Specific Skills & Movements**	
	Maximize mechanical performance to allow optimal specific skills capability		Master movements and reactions to the demands of sport	
	Muscular Development III *Heavy Power*	Fortify	**Anaerobic Expansion**	
	Maximize connective tissue excitability and efficiency		Expand upon anaerobic capacity by implementing high intensity repetitions	
	Muscular Development II *Hypertrophy*		**Aerobic Capacity**	
	A hybrid between Muscular Development I & II		Improve the capacity at which oxygen can get to working muscles	
	Muscular Development I *Muscular Endurance*		**Threshold Development**	
	Increase the performance of metabolic pathways associated with repetitive muscle contraction		Establish resistance to fatigue at the ventilitory/lactic threshold	
	Functional Stability & Neuromuscular Efficiency	Prepare	**Aerobic Elevation**	
	Improve motor control		Introduce aerobic elevation strategies to raise ventilitory threshold, increasing aerobic capacity	
	Basic Mobility & Corrective Strategies	Learn	**Metabolic Stimulation**	
	Work on any muscle imbalances & joint dysfunctions		Elevate heart rate in a novice & non-sports specific manner	
Mental Foundation & Support Structure				
Motivation | Dedication | Resources				

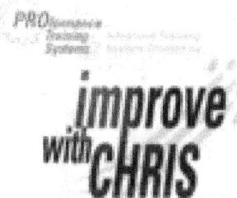

A system is an adapting method for performing a task. Whereas a program is fixed, a system changes with the individual. This system consists of two domains: Mechanical, which is composed of muscles, bones, tendons, ligaments, fascia, etc.; and Metabolic, which consist of energy systems, cardiovascular and cardiopulmonary development, etc. Both of these domains advance up the model in themes, Learn, Prepare, Fortify, and Potential. The mission of the progression model is to advance human control and capacity to its upper limit by transcending and unifying the body mechanically and metabolically while taking into account the individual's mental commitment and social support. The main goal is to mold the athlete into their potential self. The first theme is Learn. This is where basic mechanical mobility is re-taught to the individual so they are capable of using correct movement patterns during later development. We are all born with proper movements patterns; developing them as we age through trial and error. We lose the ability to perform these patterns correctly as we get older and lazier. This is a result of our body's natural desire to become more efficient. We take "movement shortcuts" to make motion more efficient, resulting in poor movement patterns and increased risk of injury. By undergoing corrective exercise strategies and basic mobility drills it re-establishes these movement patterns within the athlete, setting them up for success as they progress through the following themes. Metabolic stimulation is also introduced during the learning theme. Here the body becomes re- acquainted with an elevated heart rate in a fitness setting. This is accomplished by participating in non- sports specific activities. It is important to think of the learning theme not as exercise but as priming the body for exercise in the following themes. Preparing the body for advance development is the second theme. Mechanically, this takes place after efficient mobility is achieved, but before muscular development training begins. Adequate mobility and sufficient stability must be in place before focusing on developing the musculature. If the body cannot move through a full range of motion and control those movements, the athlete is not prepared to undergo performance training. During this time the athlete is performing functional stability and neuromuscular efficiency exercises to increase their bodily control in order to achieve acceptable levels of motion for the fortify stage. Metabolically, the body is being introduced to steady state cardio in order to elevate its aerobic capacity. By elevating aerobic capacity it raises the anaerobic threshold, this makes aerobic elevation valuable for endurance and non-endurance sports. Fortification is the third theme of advancement. Here muscular development strategies are introduced during mechanical training in order to improve the muscle fiber's energy systems and power development potential. This is accomplished over a period of three stages. Muscular Endurance, when the focus is on increasing the performance of metabolic pathways associated with repetitive muscle contractions. Muscular Hypertrophy, which is a blend of muscular endurance and strength development. The third stage, Heavy Power focuses on maximizing connective tissue excitability and efficiency. On the metabolic side of the coin, Threshold Development, which is elevating your body's ventilatory threshold and lactate tolerance, is implemented through ventilatory and lactic threshold training. Threshold development training fortifies the body against fatigue while performing at the ventilatory/ lactic threshold. This allows the athlete to last longer at a higher work rate than their competition. Once the threshold is fortified, Aerobic Capacity is established by improving the capacity at which oxygen can get to working muscles. High intensity training done at VO2max will help the muscles extract more oxygen from the blood stream during high intensity competition. The final metabolic fortification stage is Anaerobic Expansion, which expands upon anaerobic capacity by implementing high intensity anaerobic repetitions. Anaerobic expansion is vital for reaching full athletic potential. Even a distance athlete undergoes anaerobic metabolism as acidosis accumulates in their legs. Furthermore, the adaptations that occur during anaerobic expansion activities are a necessary primer for the demands of the potential theme. The final theme is Potential, and it is here that athletes reach their athletic potential. Mechanically this is accomplished through advanced movement systems consisting of power and maximum functional movement integration at full speed (training form drills). It is this stage of training that has the highest functional carryover to sport. Metabolically, this entails mastering movements and reactions to the demands of sport. These reactions can be movements or physiological demands. The ultimate goal of the potential theme is to unite the mechanical and metabolic components into one hybrid training method where the athlete can reach their potential. That said, it is important to note that just because one has reached a theme of the model, it does not mean that they cannot regress back to a prior theme due to lack of training or poor training effort. Progress is determined through constant evaluation and systems adaptation to that evaluation. If the athlete does not pass the evaluation, then the system adapts to his needs. Moreover, since the individual is training their body for specific movements and physiological demands, it is vital that we treat the body as a whole movement system rather than a series of independent movements. The human movement system works as a whole so the model is meant to train the body using the most highly integrated functional movements applicable to each theme.

Additionally, once the goals of one theme are accomplished that theme is not forgotten as we progress up the hierarchy. The skills learned and abilities acquired are present in the integrated functional movements at the next level. All of the traits and demands of the previous theme are present in the next one. This lessens the chance of re-occurrence of a mechanical limitation or metabolic detraining. Finally, but perhaps most important is the Mental Foundation and Support Structure of PROformance Training Systems; motivation, dedication, and resources. Athletes need to have motivation towards their goal if they are going to be dedicated to the extent necessary to reach their true potential. Tremendous amounts of dedication in the form of commitment and consistency must be present if the athlete expects to adapt and progress up the themes. Constant mental sport coaching is a core element of a strong mental foundation. Moreover, adequate resources such as quality coaching, family and friend support, acceptable equipment, and ample time need to be available for the athlete to undergo their training with the least amount of road blocks. A strong mental foundation and solid support structure can consist of variable things depending on the particular athlete. Therefore, it is vital to perform a consultation and follow-up consultation with the athlete on a regular basis to make certain the needs of the foundation and structure have not changed and are still being met. PROformance Training Systems is not the only method of progressing an individual towards optimal performance. However, based on my education and experience, it is the one that I feel is the most justified and has been highly successful for my athletes.

PROformance Training Systems
Exercise Recommendation Chart

Type of Activity		Lose Ability	Maintain Ability	Gain Ability	Time (Duration)
Structural	*Metabolic*	Days Per Week (Frequency)			Minutes
Basic Mobility & Strength	Weight Control / Maintenance	1-2	3	4-5	30
Hypertrophy (Size)	Competitive Endurance	<3	3-4	5-6	45-90
Athletic Strength	Competitive Conditioning (For Non-Endurance Athletes)	1-2	3	4-5	45-60
Competitive Power	Basic Cardiovascular Health	1	2	3-4	30-45

The purpose of this chart is to show you what it takes to lose, maintain, and gain ability in specific areas of fitness.

Structural and metabolic types of activity are listed next to each other for the sole purpose of making the chart easier to read. It has nothing to do with matching up structural with metabolic training. That is beyond the scope of the chart.

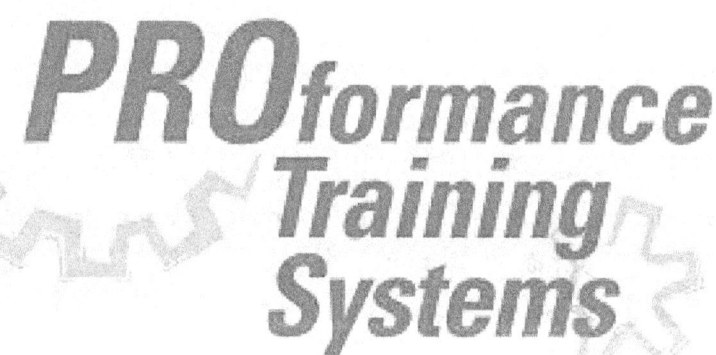

Types of activity can overlap for a given day. For instance, basic mobility and strength can be performed between sets focusing on competitive power on the same day. This allows for the best use of time while improving upon all types of activity.

Dynamic Warm up

Be sure to perform an appropriate dynamic warmup prior to engaging in any fitness activity.

#1

Activity	Sets	Reps/Dist.	Weight/Time	Rest

Dynamic Warm up

Be sure to perform an appropriate dynamic warmup prior to engaging in any fitness activity.

#2

Activity	Sets	Reps/Dist.	Weight/Time	Rest

Cool Down

Be sure to perform an appropriate cool down after any fitness activity.

#1

Activity	Sets	Reps/Dist.	Weight/Time	Rest

Cool Down

Be sure to perform an appropriate cool down after any fitness activity.

#2

Activity	Sets	Reps/Dist.	Weight/Time	Rest

Mechanical Theme

Mob. > Corr. > Fun. Stability > NM Efficiency > Musc. Endurance > Hypertrophy > Heavy Power > Max Power > A.M.S.

Metabolic Theme

Met. Stim. > Aero. Elevation > Thresh. Development > Aero. Capacity > An. Expansion > Spec. Movements > Spec. Skills

Date	Warm Up		Cool Down		Movements/ Focus Area
	Exercise	*Duration*	*Exercise*	*Duration*	
___/___/___					

Activity	Rx (reps/dist. @ weight/time)	Rest
	___@___, ___@___, ___@___, ___@___, ___@___, ___@___	
	___@___, ___@___, ___@___, ___@___, ___@___, ___@___	
	___@___, ___@___, ___@___, ___@___, ___@___, ___@___	
	___@___, ___@___, ___@___, ___@___, ___@___, ___@___	
	___@___, ___@___, ___@___, ___@___, ___@___, ___@___	
	___@___, ___@___, ___@___, ___@___, ___@___, ___@___	
	___@___, ___@___, ___@___, ___@___, ___@___, ___@___	
	___@___, ___@___, ___@___, ___@___, ___@___, ___@___	
	___@___, ___@___, ___@___, ___@___, ___@___, ___@___	
	___@___, ___@___, ___@___, ___@___, ___@___, ___@___	
	___@___, ___@___, ___@___, ___@___, ___@___, ___@___	

Mechanical Theme
Mob. > Corr. > Fun. Stability > NM Efficiency > Musc. Endurance > Hypertrophy > Heavy Power > Max Power > A.M.S.

Metabolic Theme
Met. Stim. > Aero. Elevation > Thresh. Development > Aero. Capacity > An. Expansion > Spec. Movements > Spec. Skills

Date	Warm Up		Cool Down		Movements/ Focus Area
	Exercise	*Duration*	*Exercise*	*Duration*	
___ / ___ / ___					

Activity	Rx (reps/dist. @ weight/time)	Rest
	___@___, ___@___, ___@___, ___@___, ___@___, ___@___	
	___@___, ___@___, ___@___, ___@___, ___@___, ___@___	
	___@___, ___@___, ___@___, ___@___, ___@___, ___@___	
	___@___, ___@___, ___@___, ___@___, ___@___, ___@___	
	___@___, ___@___, ___@___, ___@___, ___@___, ___@___	
	___@___, ___@___, ___@___, ___@___, ___@___, ___@___	
	___@___, ___@___, ___@___, ___@___, ___@___, ___@___	
	___@___, ___@___, ___@___, ___@___, ___@___, ___@___	
	___@___, ___@___, ___@___, ___@___, ___@___, ___@___	
	___@___, ___@___, ___@___, ___@___, ___@___, ___@___	

Mechanical Theme

Mob. > Corr. > Fun. Stability > NM Efficiency > Musc. Endurance > Hypertrophy > Heavy Power > Max Power > A.M.S.

Metabolic Theme

Met. Stim. > Aero. Elevation > Thresh. Development > Aero. Capacity > An. Expansion > Spec. Movements > Spec. Skills

Date	Warm Up		Cool Down		Movements/ Focus Area
	Exercise	*Duration*	*Exercise*	*Duration*	
___/___/___					

Activity	Rx (reps/dist. @ weight/time)	Rest
	___@___, ___@___, ___@___, ___@___, ___@___, ___@___	
	___@___, ___@___, ___@___, ___@___, ___@___, ___@___	
	___@___, ___@___, ___@___, ___@___, ___@___, ___@___	
	___@___, ___@___, ___@___, ___@___, ___@___, ___@___	
	___@___, ___@___, ___@___, ___@___, ___@___, ___@___	
	___@___, ___@___, ___@___, ___@___, ___@___, ___@___	
	___@___, ___@___, ___@___, ___@___, ___@___, ___@___	
	___@___, ___@___, ___@___, ___@___, ___@___, ___@___	
	___@___, ___@___, ___@___, ___@___, ___@___, ___@___	

Mechanical Theme
Mob. > Corr. > Fun. Stability > NM Efficiency > Musc. Endurance > Hypertrophy > Heavy Power > Max Power > A.M.S.

Metabolic Theme
Met. Stim. > Aero. Elevation > Thresh. Development > Aero. Capacity > An. Expansion > Spec. Movements > Spec. Skills

Date	Warm Up		Cool Down		Movements/ Focus Area
	Exercise	Duration	Exercise	Duration	
__ / __ / __					

Activity	Rx (reps/dist. @ weight/time)	Rest
	____@____, ____@____, ____@____,	
	____@____, ____@____, ____@____	
	____@____, ____@____, ____@____,	
	____@____, ____@____, ____@____	
	____@____, ____@____, ____@____,	
	____@____, ____@____, ____@____	
	____@____, ____@____, ____@____,	
	____@____, ____@____, ____@____	
	____@____, ____@____, ____@____,	
	____@____, ____@____, ____@____	
	____@____, ____@____, ____@____,	
	____@____, ____@____, ____@____	
	____@____, ____@____, ____@____,	
	____@____, ____@____, ____@____	
	____@____, ____@____, ____@____,	
	____@____, ____@____, ____@____	

Mechanical Theme

Mob. > Corr. > Fun. Stability > NM Efficiency > Musc. Endurance > Hypertrophy > Heavy Power > Max Power > A.M.S.

Metabolic Theme

Met. Stim. > Aero. Elevation > Thresh. Development > Aero. Capacity > An. Expansion > Spec. Movements > Spec. Skills

Date	Warm Up		Cool Down		Movements/ Focus Area
	Exercise	*Duration*	*Exercise*	*Duration*	
__/__/__					

Activity	Rx (reps/dist. @ weight/time)	Rest
	@____, ____@____, ____@____,	
	____@____, ____@____, ____@____	
	____@____, ____@____, ____@____,	
	____@____, ____@____, ____@____	
	____@____, ____@____, ____@____,	
	____@____, ____@____, ____@____	
	____@____, ____@____, ____@____,	
	____@____, ____@____, ____@____	
	____@____, ____@____, ____@____,	
	____@____, ____@____, ____@____	
	____@____, ____@____, ____@____,	
	____@____, ____@____, ____@____	
	____@____, ____@____, ____@____,	
	____@____, ____@____, ____@____	
	____@____, ____@____, ____@____,	
	____@____, ____@____, ____@____	
	____@____, ____@____, ____@____,	
	____@____, ____@____, ____@____	
	____@____, ____@____, ____@____,	
	____@____, ____@____, ____@____	

Mechanical Theme
Mob. > Corr. > Fun. Stability > NM Efficiency > Musc. Endurance > Hypertrophy > Heavy Power > Max Power > A.M.S.

Metabolic Theme
Met. Stim. > Aero. Elevation > Thresh. Development > Aero. Capacity > An. Expansion > Spec. Movements > Spec. Skills

Date	Warm Up		Cool Down		Movements/ Focus Area
	Exercise	*Duration*	*Exercise*	*Duration*	
___ / ___ / ___					

Activity	**Rx** (reps/dist. @ weight/time)	Rest
	____@____ , ____@____ , ____@____ , ____@____ , ____@____ , ____@____	
	____@____ , ____@____ , ____@____ , ____@____ , ____@____ , ____@____	
	____@____ , ____@____ , ____@____ , ____@____ , ____@____ , ____@____	
	____@____ , ____@____ , ____@____ , ____@____ , ____@____ , ____@____	
	____@____ , ____@____ , ____@____ , ____@____ , ____@____ , ____@____	
	____@____ , ____@____ , ____@____ , ____@____ , ____@____ , ____@____	
	____@____ , ____@____ , ____@____ , ____@____ , ____@____ , ____@____	
	____@____ , ____@____ , ____@____ , ____@____ , ____@____ , ____@____	
	____@____ , ____@____ , ____@____ , ____@____ , ____@____ , ____@____	
	____@____ , ____@____ , ____@____ , ____@____ , ____@____ , ____@____	

Mechanical Theme
Mob. > Corr. > Fun. Stability > NM Efficiency > Musc. Endurance > Hypertrophy > Heavy Power > Max Power > A.M.S.

Metabolic Theme
Met. Stim. > Aero. Elevation > Thresh. Development > Aero. Capacity > An. Expansion > Spec. Movements > Spec. Skills

Date	Warm Up		Cool Down		Movements/ Focus Area
	Exercise	*Duration*	*Exercise*	*Duration*	
___/___/___					

Activity	Rx (reps/dist. @ weight/time)	Rest
	___@___, ___@___, ___@___,	
	___@___, ___@___, ___@___	
	___@___, ___@___, ___@___,	
	___@___, ___@___, ___@___	
	___@___, ___@___, ___@___,	
	___@___, ___@___, ___@___	
	___@___, ___@___, ___@___,	
	___@___, ___@___, ___@___	
	___@___, ___@___, ___@___,	
	___@___, ___@___, ___@___	
	___@___, ___@___, ___@___,	
	___@___, ___@___, ___@___	
	___@___, ___@___, ___@___,	
	___@___, ___@___, ___@___	
	___@___, ___@___, ___@___,	
	___@___, ___@___, ___@___	
	___@___, ___@___, ___@___,	
	___@___, ___@___, ___@___	
	___@___, ___@___, ___@___,	
	___@___, ___@___, ___@___	

Mechanical Theme
Mob. > Corr. > Fun. Stability > NM Efficiency > Musc. Endurance > Hypertrophy > Heavy Power > Max Power > A.M.S.

Metabolic Theme
Met. Stim. > Aero. Elevation > Thresh. Development > Aero. Capacity > An. Expansion > Spec. Movements > Spec. Skills

Date	Warm Up		Cool Down		Movements/ Focus Area
	Exercise	*Duration*	*Exercise*	*Duration*	
___/___/___					

Activity	Rx (reps/dist. @ weight/time)	Rest
	____@____, ____@____, ____@____, ____@____, ____@____, ____@____	
	____@____, ____@____, ____@____, ____@____, ____@____, ____@____	
	____@____, ____@____, ____@____, ____@____, ____@____, ____@____	
	____@____, ____@____, ____@____, ____@____, ____@____, ____@____	
	____@____, ____@____, ____@____, ____@____, ____@____, ____@____	
	____@____, ____@____, ____@____, ____@____, ____@____, ____@____	
	____@____, ____@____, ____@____, ____@____, ____@____, ____@____	
	____@____, ____@____, ____@____, ____@____, ____@____, ____@____	
	____@____, ____@____, ____@____, ____@____, ____@____, ____@____	
	____@____, ____@____, ____@____, ____@____, ____@____, ____@____	
	____@____, ____@____, ____@____, ____@____, ____@____, ____@____	

Mechanical Theme

Mob. > Corr. > Fun. Stability > NM Efficiency > Musc. Endurance > Hypertrophy > Heavy Power > Max Power > A.M.S.

Metabolic Theme

Met. Stim. > Aero. Elevation > Thresh. Development > Aero. Capacity > An. Expansion > Spec. Movements > Spec. Skills

Date	Warm Up		Cool Down		Movements/ Focus Area
	Exercise	*Duration*	*Exercise*	*Duration*	
__/__/__					

Activity	Rx (reps/dist. @ weight/time)	Rest
	___@___, ___@___, ___@___,	
	___@___, ___@___, ___@___	
	___@___, ___@___, ___@___,	
	___@___, ___@___, ___@___	
	___@___, ___@___, ___@___,	
	___@___, ___@___, ___@___	
	___@___, ___@___, ___@___,	
	___@___, ___@___, ___@___	
	___@___, ___@___, ___@___,	
	___@___, ___@___, ___@___	
	___@___, ___@___, ___@___,	
	___@___, ___@___, ___@___	
	___@___, ___@___, ___@___,	
	___@___, ___@___, ___@___	
	___@___, ___@___, ___@___,	
	___@___, ___@___, ___@___	
	___@___, ___@___, ___@___,	
	___@___, ___@___, ___@___	
	___@___, ___@___, ___@___,	
	___@___, ___@___, ___@___	
	___@___, ___@___, ___@___,	
	___@___, ___@___, ___@___	

Mechanical Theme
Mob. > Corr. > Fun. Stability > NM Efficiency > Musc. Endurance > Hypertrophy > Heavy Power > Max Power > A.M.S.

Metabolic Theme
Met. Stim. > Aero. Elevation > Thresh. Development > Aero. Capacity > An. Expansion > Spec. Movements > Spec. Skills

Date	Warm Up		Cool Down		Movements/ Focus Area
	Exercise	*Duration*	*Exercise*	*Duration*	
___/___/___					

Activity	Rx (reps/dist. @ weight/time)	Rest
	___@___, ___@___, ___@___, ___@___, ___@___, ___@___	
	___@___, ___@___, ___@___, ___@___, ___@___, ___@___	
	___@___, ___@___, ___@___, ___@___, ___@___, ___@___	
	___@___, ___@___, ___@___, ___@___, ___@___, ___@___	
	___@___, ___@___, ___@___, ___@___, ___@___, ___@___	
	___@___, ___@___, ___@___, ___@___, ___@___, ___@___	
	___@___, ___@___, ___@___, ___@___, ___@___, ___@___	
	___@___, ___@___, ___@___, ___@___, ___@___, ___@___	
	___@___, ___@___, ___@___, ___@___, ___@___, ___@___	
	___@___, ___@___, ___@___, ___@___, ___@___, ___@___	

Mechanical Theme

Mob. > Corr. > Fun. Stability > NM Efficiency > Musc. Endurance > Hypertrophy > Heavy Power > Max Power > A.M.S.

Metabolic Theme

Met. Stim. > Aero. Elevation > Thresh. Development > Aero. Capacity > An. Expansion > Spec. Movements > Spec. Skills

Date	Warm Up		Cool Down		Movements/ Focus Area
	Exercise	*Duration*	*Exercise*	*Duration*	
___ / ___ / ___					

Activity	Rx (reps/dist. @ weight/time)	Rest
	____@____ , ____@____ , ____@____ ,	
	____@____ , ____@____ , ____@____	
	____@____ , ____@____ , ____@____ ,	
	____@____ , ____@____ , ____@____	
	____@____ , ____@____ , ____@____ ,	
	____@____ , ____@____ , ____@____	
	____@____ , ____@____ , ____@____ ,	
	____@____ , ____@____ , ____@____	
	____@____ , ____@____ , ____@____ ,	
	____@____ , ____@____ , ____@____	
	____@____ , ____@____ , ____@____ ,	
	____@____ , ____@____ , ____@____	
	____@____ , ____@____ , ____@____ ,	
	____@____ , ____@____ , ____@____	
	____@____ , ____@____ , ____@____ ,	
	____@____ , ____@____ , ____@____	
	____@____ , ____@____ , ____@____ ,	
	____@____ , ____@____ , ____@____	
	____@____ , ____@____ , ____@____ ,	
	____@____ , ____@____ , ____@____	

Mechanical Theme
Mob. > Corr. > Fun. Stability > NM Efficiency > Musc. Endurance > Hypertrophy > Heavy Power > Max Power > A.M.S.

Metabolic Theme
Met. Stim. > Aero. Elevation > Thresh. Development > Aero. Capacity > An. Expansion > Spec. Movements > Spec. Skills

Date	Warm Up		Cool Down		Movements/ Focus Area
	Exercise	*Duration*	*Exercise*	*Duration*	
___/___/___					

Activity	**Rx** (reps/dist. @ weight/time)	Rest
	____@____, ____@____, ____@____, ____@____, ____@____, ____@____	
	____@____, ____@____, ____@____, ____@____, ____@____, ____@____	
	____@____, ____@____, ____@____, ____@____, ____@____, ____@____	
	____@____, ____@____, ____@____, ____@____, ____@____, ____@____	
	____@____, ____@____, ____@____, ____@____, ____@____, ____@____	
	____@____, ____@____, ____@____, ____@____, ____@____, ____@____	
	____@____, ____@____, ____@____, ____@____, ____@____, ____@____	
	____@____, ____@____, ____@____, ____@____, ____@____, ____@____	
	____@____, ____@____, ____@____, ____@____, ____@____, ____@____	
	____@____, ____@____, ____@____, ____@____, ____@____, ____@____	
	____@____, ____@____, ____@____, ____@____, ____@____, ____@____	

Mechanical Theme
Mob. > Corr. > Fun. Stability > NM Efficiency > Musc. Endurance > Hypertrophy > Heavy Power > Max Power > A.M.S.

Metabolic Theme
Met. Stim. > Aero. Elevation > Thresh. Development > Aero. Capacity > An. Expansion > Spec. Movements > Spec. Skills

Date	Warm Up		Cool Down		Movements/ Focus Area
	Exercise	*Duration*	*Exercise*	*Duration*	
___/___/___					

Activity	Rx (reps/dist. @ weight/time)	Rest
	____@____, ____@____, ____@____,	
	____@____, ____@____, ____@____	
	____@____, ____@____, ____@____,	
	____@____, ____@____, ____@____	
	____@____, ____@____, ____@____,	
	____@____, ____@____, ____@____	
	____@____, ____@____, ____@____,	
	____@____, ____@____, ____@____	
	____@____, ____@____, ____@____,	
	____@____, ____@____, ____@____	
	____@____, ____@____, ____@____,	
	____@____, ____@____, ____@____	
	____@____, ____@____, ____@____,	
	____@____, ____@____, ____@____	
	____@____, ____@____, ____@____,	
	____@____, ____@____, ____@____	
	____@____, ____@____, ____@____,	
	____@____, ____@____, ____@____	
	____@____, ____@____, ____@____,	
	____@____, ____@____, ____@____	

27

Mechanical Theme
Mob. > Corr. > Fun. Stability > NM Efficiency > Musc. Endurance > Hypertrophy > Heavy Power > Max Power > A.M.S.

Metabolic Theme
Met. Stim. > Aero. Elevation > Thresh. Development > Aero. Capacity > An. Expansion > Spec. Movements > Spec. Skills

Date	Warm Up		Cool Down		Movements/ Focus Area
	Exercise	*Duration*	*Exercise*	*Duration*	
___/___/___					

Activity	Rx (reps/dist. @ weight/time)	Rest
	____@____, ____@____, ____@____, ____@____, ____@____, ____@____	
	____@____, ____@____, ____@____, ____@____, ____@____, ____@____	
	____@____, ____@____, ____@____, ____@____, ____@____, ____@____	
	____@____, ____@____, ____@____, ____@____, ____@____, ____@____	
	____@____, ____@____, ____@____, ____@____, ____@____, ____@____	
	____@____, ____@____, ____@____, ____@____, ____@____, ____@____	
	____@____, ____@____, ____@____, ____@____, ____@____, ____@____	
	____@____, ____@____, ____@____, ____@____, ____@____, ____@____	
	____@____, ____@____, ____@____, ____@____, ____@____, ____@____	
	____@____, ____@____, ____@____, ____@____, ____@____, ____@____	

Mechanical Theme
Mob. > Corr. > Fun. Stability > NM Efficiency > Musc. Endurance > Hypertrophy > Heavy Power > Max Power > A.M.S.

Metabolic Theme
Met. Stim. > Aero. Elevation > Thresh. Development > Aero. Capacity > An. Expansion > Spec. Movements > Spec. Skills

Date	Warm Up		Cool Down		Movements/ Focus Area
	Exercise	*Duration*	*Exercise*	*Duration*	
___/___/___					

Activity	Rx (reps/dist. @ weight/time)	Rest
	___@___, ___@___, ___@___,	
	___@___, ___@___, ___@___	
	___@___, ___@___, ___@___,	
	___@___, ___@___, ___@___	
	___@___, ___@___, ___@___,	
	___@___, ___@___, ___@___	
	___@___, ___@___, ___@___,	
	___@___, ___@___, ___@___	
	___@___, ___@___, ___@___,	
	___@___, ___@___, ___@___	
	___@___, ___@___, ___@___,	
	___@___, ___@___, ___@___	
	___@___, ___@___, ___@___,	
	___@___, ___@___, ___@___	
	___@___, ___@___, ___@___,	
	___@___, ___@___, ___@___	
	___@___, ___@___, ___@___,	
	___@___, ___@___, ___@___	
	___@___, ___@___, ___@___,	
	___@___, ___@___, ___@___	

Mechanical Theme
Mob. > Corr. > Fun. Stability > NM Efficiency > Musc. Endurance > Hypertrophy > Heavy Power > Max Power > A.M.S.

Metabolic Theme
Met. Stim. > Aero. Elevation > Thresh. Development > Aero. Capacity > An. Expansion > Spec. Movements > Spec. Skills

Date	Warm Up		Cool Down		Movements/ Focus Area
	Exercise	*Duration*	*Exercise*	*Duration*	
___ / ___ / ___					

Activity	Rx (reps/dist. @ weight/time)	Rest
	____@____ , ____@____ , ____@____ , ____@____ , ____@____ , ____@____	
	____@____ , ____@____ , ____@____ , ____@____ , ____@____ , ____@____	
	____@____ , ____@____ , ____@____ , ____@____ , ____@____ , ____@____	
	____@____ , ____@____ , ____@____ , ____@____ , ____@____ , ____@____	
	____@____ , ____@____ , ____@____ , ____@____ , ____@____ , ____@____	
	____@____ , ____@____ , ____@____ , ____@____ , ____@____ , ____@____	
	____@____ , ____@____ , ____@____ , ____@____ , ____@____ , ____@____	
	____@____ , ____@____ , ____@____ , ____@____ , ____@____ , ____@____	
	____@____ , ____@____ , ____@____ , ____@____ , ____@____ , ____@____	
	____@____ , ____@____ , ____@____ , ____@____ , ____@____ , ____@____	
	____@____ , ____@____ , ____@____ , ____@____ , ____@____ , ____@____	

Mechanical Theme
Mob. > Corr. > Fun. Stability > NM Efficiency > Musc. Endurance > Hypertrophy > Heavy Power > Max Power > A.M.S.

Metabolic Theme
Met. Stim. > Aero. Elevation > Thresh. Development > Aero. Capacity > An. Expansion > Spec. Movements > Spec. Skills

Date	Warm Up		Cool Down		Movements/ Focus Area
	Exercise	*Duration*	*Exercise*	*Duration*	
___/___/___					

Activity	Rx (reps/dist. @ weight/time)	Rest
	___@___, ___@___, ___@___,	
	___@___, ___@___, ___@___	
	___@___, ___@___, ___@___,	
	___@___, ___@___, ___@___	
	___@___, ___@___, ___@___,	
	___@___, ___@___, ___@___	
	___@___, ___@___, ___@___,	
	___@___, ___@___, ___@___	
	___@___, ___@___, ___@___,	
	___@___, ___@___, ___@___	
	___@___, ___@___, ___@___,	
	___@___, ___@___, ___@___	
	___@___, ___@___, ___@___,	
	___@___, ___@___, ___@___	
	___@___, ___@___, ___@___,	
	___@___, ___@___, ___@___	
	___@___, ___@___, ___@___,	
	___@___, ___@___, ___@___	
	___@___, ___@___, ___@___,	
	___@___, ___@___, ___@___	

Mechanical Theme
Mob. > Corr. > Fun. Stability > NM Efficiency > Musc. Endurance > Hypertrophy > Heavy Power > Max Power > A.M.S.

Metabolic Theme
Met. Stim. > Aero. Elevation > Thresh. Development > Aero. Capacity > An. Expansion > Spec. Movements > Spec. Skills

Date	Warm Up		Cool Down		Movements/ Focus Area
	Exercise	*Duration*	*Exercise*	*Duration*	
___ / ___ / ___					

Activity	Rx (reps/dist. @ weight/time)	Rest
	____@____, ____@____, ____@____, ____@____, ____@____, ____@____	
	____@____, ____@____, ____@____, ____@____, ____@____, ____@____	
	____@____, ____@____, ____@____, ____@____, ____@____, ____@____	
	____@____, ____@____, ____@____, ____@____, ____@____, ____@____	
	____@____, ____@____, ____@____, ____@____, ____@____, ____@____	
	____@____, ____@____, ____@____, ____@____, ____@____, ____@____	
	____@____, ____@____, ____@____, ____@____, ____@____, ____@____	
	____@____, ____@____, ____@____, ____@____, ____@____, ____@____	
	____@____, ____@____, ____@____, ____@____, ____@____, ____@____	
	____@____, ____@____, ____@____, ____@____, ____@____, ____@____	

<table>
<tr><td colspan="5" align="center">**Mechanical Theme**</td></tr>
<tr><td colspan="5" align="center">Mob. > Corr. > Fun. Stability > NM Efficiency > Musc. Endurance > Hypertrophy > Heavy Power > Max Power > A.M.S.</td></tr>
<tr><td colspan="5" align="center">**Metabolic Theme**</td></tr>
<tr><td colspan="5" align="center">Met. Stim. > Aero. Elevation > Thresh. Development > Aero. Capacity > An. Expansion > Spec. Movements > Spec. Skills</td></tr>
<tr><td>**Date**</td><td colspan="2" align="center">**Warm Up**</td><td colspan="2" align="center">**Cool Down**</td><td>**Movements/ Focus Area**</td></tr>
</table>

Date	Warm Up		Cool Down		Movements/ Focus Area
	Exercise	*Duration*	*Exercise*	*Duration*	
___/___/___					

Activity	Rx (reps/dist. @ weight/time)	Rest
	____@____, ____@____, ____@____,	
	____@____, ____@____, ____@____	
	____@____, ____@____, ____@____,	
	____@____, ____@____, ____@____	
	____@____, ____@____, ____@____,	
	____@____, ____@____, ____@____	
	____@____, ____@____, ____@____,	
	____@____, ____@____, ____@____	
	____@____, ____@____, ____@____,	
	____@____, ____@____, ____@____	
	____@____, ____@____, ____@____,	
	____@____, ____@____, ____@____	
	____@____, ____@____, ____@____,	
	____@____, ____@____, ____@____	
	____@____, ____@____, ____@____,	
	____@____, ____@____, ____@____	
	____@____, ____@____, ____@____,	
	____@____, ____@____, ____@____	
	____@____, ____@____, ____@____,	
	____@____, ____@____, ____@____	
	____@____, ____@____, ____@____,	
	____@____, ____@____, ____@____	

Mechanical Theme
Mob. > Corr. > Fun. Stability > NM Efficiency > Musc. Endurance > Hypertrophy > Heavy Power > Max Power > A.M.S.

Metabolic Theme
Met. Stim. > Aero. Elevation > Thresh. Development > Aero. Capacity > An. Expansion > Spec. Movements > Spec. Skills

Date	Warm Up		Cool Down		Movements/ Focus Area
	Exercise	*Duration*	*Exercise*	*Duration*	
___/___/___					

Activity	**Rx** (reps/dist. @ weight/time)	Rest
	____@____, ____@____, ____@____, ____@____, ____@____, ____@____	
	____@____, ____@____, ____@____, ____@____, ____@____, ____@____	
	____@____, ____@____, ____@____, ____@____, ____@____, ____@____	
	____@____, ____@____, ____@____, ____@____, ____@____, ____@____	
	____@____, ____@____, ____@____, ____@____, ____@____, ____@____	
	____@____, ____@____, ____@____, ____@____, ____@____, ____@____	
	____@____, ____@____, ____@____, ____@____, ____@____, ____@____	
	____@____, ____@____, ____@____, ____@____, ____@____, ____@____	
	____@____, ____@____, ____@____, ____@____, ____@____, ____@____	
	____@____, ____@____, ____@____, ____@____, ____@____, ____@____	
	____@____, ____@____, ____@____, ____@____, ____@____, ____@____	

Mechanical Theme
Mob. > Corr. > Fun. Stability > NM Efficiency > Musc. Endurance > Hypertrophy > Heavy Power > Max Power > A.M.S.

Metabolic Theme
Met. Stim. > Aero. Elevation > Thresh. Development > Aero. Capacity > An. Expansion > Spec. Movements > Spec. Skills

Date	Warm Up		Cool Down		Movements/ Focus Area
	Exercise	*Duration*	*Exercise*	*Duration*	
___/___/___					

Activity	Rx (reps/dist. @ weight/time)	Rest
	___@___, ___@___, ___@___,	
	___@___, ___@___, ___@___	
	___@___, ___@___, ___@___,	
	___@___, ___@___, ___@___	
	___@___, ___@___, ___@___,	
	___@___, ___@___, ___@___	
	___@___, ___@___, ___@___,	
	___@___, ___@___, ___@___	
	___@___, ___@___, ___@___,	
	___@___, ___@___, ___@___	
	___@___, ___@___, ___@___,	
	___@___, ___@___, ___@___	
	___@___, ___@___, ___@___,	
	___@___, ___@___, ___@___	
	___@___, ___@___, ___@___,	
	___@___, ___@___, ___@___	
	___@___, ___@___, ___@___,	
	___@___, ___@___, ___@___	
	___@___, ___@___, ___@___,	
	___@___, ___@___, ___@___	
	___@___, ___@___, ___@___,	
	___@___, ___@___, ___@___	

Mechanical Theme
Mob. > Corr. > Fun. Stability > NM Efficiency > Musc. Endurance > Hypertrophy > Heavy Power > Max Power > A.M.S.

Metabolic Theme
Met. Stim. > Aero. Elevation > Thresh. Development > Aero. Capacity > An. Expansion > Spec. Movements > Spec. Skills

Date	Warm Up		Cool Down		Movements/ Focus Area
	Exercise	*Duration*	*Exercise*	*Duration*	
___ / ___ / ___					

Activity	Rx (reps/dist. @ weight/time)	Rest
	____@____, ____@____, ____@____, ____@____, ____@____, ____@____	
	____@____, ____@____, ____@____, ____@____, ____@____, ____@____	
	____@____, ____@____, ____@____, ____@____, ____@____, ____@____	
	____@____, ____@____, ____@____, ____@____, ____@____, ____@____	
	____@____, ____@____, ____@____, ____@____, ____@____, ____@____	
	____@____, ____@____, ____@____, ____@____, ____@____, ____@____	
	____@____, ____@____, ____@____, ____@____, ____@____, ____@____	
	____@____, ____@____, ____@____, ____@____, ____@____, ____@____	
	____@____, ____@____, ____@____, ____@____, ____@____, ____@____	
	____@____, ____@____, ____@____, ____@____, ____@____, ____@____	

Mechanical Theme
Mob. > Corr. > Fun. Stability > NM Efficiency > Musc. Endurance > Hypertrophy > Heavy Power > Max Power > A.M.S.

Metabolic Theme
Met. Stim. > Aero. Elevation > Thresh. Development > Aero. Capacity > An. Expansion > Spec. Movements > Spec. Skills

Date	Warm Up		Cool Down		Movements/ Focus Area
	Exercise	*Duration*	*Exercise*	*Duration*	
___ / ___ / ___					

Activity	**Rx** (reps/dist. @ weight/time)	Rest
	___@___ , ___@___ , ___@___ ,	
	___@___ , ___@___ , ___@___	
	___@___ , ___@___ , ___@___ ,	
	___@___ , ___@___ , ___@___	
	___@___ , ___@___ , ___@___ ,	
	___@___ , ___@___ , ___@___	
	___@___ , ___@___ , ___@___ ,	
	___@___ , ___@___ , ___@___	
	___@___ , ___@___ , ___@___ ,	
	___@___ , ___@___ , ___@___	
	___@___ , ___@___ , ___@___ ,	
	___@___ , ___@___ , ___@___	
	___@___ , ___@___ , ___@___ ,	
	___@___ , ___@___ , ___@___	
	___@___ , ___@___ , ___@___ ,	
	___@___ , ___@___ , ___@___	
	___@___ , ___@___ , ___@___ ,	
	___@___ , ___@___ , ___@___	
	___@___ , ___@___ , ___@___ ,	
	___@___ , ___@___ , ___@___	

Mechanical Theme
Mob. > Corr. > Fun. Stability > NM Efficiency > Musc. Endurance > Hypertrophy > Heavy Power > Max Power > A.M.S.

Metabolic Theme
Met. Stim. > Aero. Elevation > Thresh. Development > Aero. Capacity > An. Expansion > Spec. Movements > Spec. Skills

Date	Warm Up		Cool Down		Movements/ Focus Area
	Exercise	*Duration*	*Exercise*	*Duration*	
___/___/___					

Activity	Rx (reps/dist. @ weight/time)	Rest
	____@____, ____@____, ____@____, ____@____, ____@____, ____@____	
	____@____, ____@____, ____@____, ____@____, ____@____, ____@____	
	____@____, ____@____, ____@____, ____@____, ____@____, ____@____	
	____@____, ____@____, ____@____, ____@____, ____@____, ____@____	
	____@____, ____@____, ____@____, ____@____, ____@____, ____@____	
	____@____, ____@____, ____@____, ____@____, ____@____, ____@____	
	____@____, ____@____, ____@____, ____@____, ____@____, ____@____	
	____@____, ____@____, ____@____, ____@____, ____@____, ____@____	
	____@____, ____@____, ____@____, ____@____, ____@____, ____@____	
	____@____, ____@____, ____@____, ____@____, ____@____, ____@____	

Mechanical Theme
Mob. > Corr. > Fun. Stability > NM Efficiency > Musc. Endurance > Hypertrophy > Heavy Power > Max Power > A.M.S.

Metabolic Theme
Met. Stim. > Aero. Elevation > Thresh. Development > Aero. Capacity > An. Expansion > Spec. Movements > Spec. Skills

Date	Warm Up		Cool Down		Movements/ Focus Area
	Exercise	*Duration*	*Exercise*	*Duration*	
___/___/___					

Activity	Rx (reps/dist. @ weight/time)	Rest
	____@____, ____@____, ____@____,	
	____@____, ____@____, ____@____	
	____@____, ____@____, ____@____,	
	____@____, ____@____, ____@____	
	____@____, ____@____, ____@____,	
	____@____, ____@____, ____@____	
	____@____, ____@____, ____@____,	
	____@____, ____@____, ____@____	
	____@____, ____@____, ____@____,	
	____@____, ____@____, ____@____	
	____@____, ____@____, ____@____,	
	____@____, ____@____, ____@____	
	____@____, ____@____, ____@____,	
	____@____, ____@____, ____@____	
	____@____, ____@____, ____@____,	
	____@____, ____@____, ____@____	
	____@____, ____@____, ____@____,	
	____@____, ____@____, ____@____	
	____@____, ____@____, ____@____,	
	____@____, ____@____, ____@____	

Mechanical Theme
Mob. > Corr. > Fun. Stability > NM Efficiency > Musc. Endurance > Hypertrophy > Heavy Power > Max Power > A.M.S.

Metabolic Theme
Met. Stim. > Aero. Elevation > Thresh. Development > Aero. Capacity > An. Expansion > Spec. Movements > Spec. Skills

Date	Warm Up		Cool Down		Movements/ Focus Area
	Exercise	*Duration*	*Exercise*	*Duration*	
___/___/___					

Activity	Rx (reps/dist. @ weight/time)	Rest
	____@____, ____@____, ____@____,	
	____@____, ____@____, ____@____	
	____@____, ____@____, ____@____,	
	____@____, ____@____, ____@____	
	____@____, ____@____, ____@____,	
	____@____, ____@____, ____@____	
	____@____, ____@____, ____@____,	
	____@____, ____@____, ____@____	
	____@____, ____@____, ____@____,	
	____@____, ____@____, ____@____	
	____@____, ____@____, ____@____,	
	____@____, ____@____, ____@____	
	____@____, ____@____, ____@____,	
	____@____, ____@____, ____@____	
	____@____, ____@____, ____@____,	
	____@____, ____@____, ____@____	
	____@____, ____@____, ____@____,	
	____@____, ____@____, ____@____	

Mechanical Theme
Mob. > Corr. > Fun. Stability > NM Efficiency > Musc. Endurance > Hypertrophy > Heavy Power > Max Power > A.M.S.

Metabolic Theme
Met. Stim. > Aero. Elevation > Thresh. Development > Aero. Capacity > An. Expansion > Spec. Movements > Spec. Skills

Date	Warm Up		Cool Down		Movements/ Focus Area
	Exercise	*Duration*	*Exercise*	*Duration*	
___ / ___ / ___					

Activity	Rx (reps/dist. @ weight/time)	Rest
	____@____, ____@____, ____@____,	
	____@____, ____@____, ____@____	
	____@____, ____@____, ____@____,	
	____@____, ____@____, ____@____	
	____@____, ____@____, ____@____,	
	____@____, ____@____, ____@____	
	____@____, ____@____, ____@____,	
	____@____, ____@____, ____@____	
	____@____, ____@____, ____@____,	
	____@____, ____@____, ____@____	
	____@____, ____@____, ____@____,	
	____@____, ____@____, ____@____	
	____@____, ____@____, ____@____,	
	____@____, ____@____, ____@____	
	____@____, ____@____, ____@____,	
	____@____, ____@____, ____@____	
	____@____, ____@____, ____@____,	
	____@____, ____@____, ____@____	
	____@____, ____@____, ____@____,	
	____@____, ____@____, ____@____	
	____@____, ____@____, ____@____,	
	____@____, ____@____, ____@____	

Mechanical Theme
Mob. > Corr. > Fun. Stability > NM Efficiency > Musc. Endurance > Hypertrophy > Heavy Power > Max Power > A.M.S.

Metabolic Theme
Met. Stim. > Aero. Elevation > Thresh. Development > Aero. Capacity > An. Expansion > Spec. Movements > Spec. Skills

Date	Warm Up		Cool Down		Movements/ Focus Area
	Exercise	*Duration*	*Exercise*	*Duration*	
___/___/___					

Activity	**Rx** (reps/dist. @ weight/time)	Rest
	____@____, ____@____, ____@____, ____@____, ____@____, ____@____	
	____@____, ____@____, ____@____, ____@____, ____@____, ____@____	
	____@____, ____@____, ____@____, ____@____, ____@____, ____@____	
	____@____, ____@____, ____@____, ____@____, ____@____, ____@____	
	____@____, ____@____, ____@____, ____@____, ____@____, ____@____	
	____@____, ____@____, ____@____, ____@____, ____@____, ____@____	
	____@____, ____@____, ____@____, ____@____, ____@____, ____@____	
	____@____, ____@____, ____@____, ____@____, ____@____, ____@____	
	____@____, ____@____, ____@____, ____@____, ____@____, ____@____	
	____@____, ____@____, ____@____, ____@____, ____@____, ____@____	
	____@____, ____@____, ____@____, ____@____, ____@____, ____@____	

Mechanical Theme
Mob. > Corr. > Fun. Stability > NM Efficiency > Musc. Endurance > Hypertrophy > Heavy Power > Max Power > A.M.S.

Metabolic Theme
Met. Stim. > Aero. Elevation > Thresh. Development > Aero. Capacity > An. Expansion > Spec. Movements > Spec. Skills

Date	Warm Up		Cool Down		Movements/ Focus Area
	Exercise	*Duration*	*Exercise*	*Duration*	
___/___/___					

Activity	Rx (reps/dist. @ weight/time)	Rest
	___@___, ___@___, ___@___,	
	___@___, ___@___, ___@___	
	___@___, ___@___, ___@___,	
	___@___, ___@___, ___@___	
	___@___, ___@___, ___@___,	
	___@___, ___@___, ___@___	
	___@___, ___@___, ___@___,	
	___@___, ___@___, ___@___	
	___@___, ___@___, ___@___,	
	___@___, ___@___, ___@___	
	___@___, ___@___, ___@___,	
	___@___, ___@___, ___@___	
	___@___, ___@___, ___@___,	
	___@___, ___@___, ___@___	
	___@___, ___@___, ___@___,	
	___@___, ___@___, ___@___	
	___@___, ___@___, ___@___,	
	___@___, ___@___, ___@___	
	___@___, ___@___, ___@___,	
	___@___, ___@___, ___@___	
	___@___, ___@___, ___@___,	
	___@___, ___@___, ___@___	

Mechanical Theme
Mob. > Corr. > Fun. Stability > NM Efficiency > Musc. Endurance > Hypertrophy > Heavy Power > Max Power > A.M.S.

Metabolic Theme
Met. Stim. > Aero. Elevation > Thresh. Development > Aero. Capacity > An. Expansion > Spec. Movements > Spec. Skills

Date	Warm Up		Cool Down		Movements/ Focus Area
	Exercise	*Duration*	*Exercise*	*Duration*	
___/___/___					

Activity	Rx (reps/dist. @ weight/time)	Rest
	___@___, ___@___, ___@___, ___@___, ___@___, ___@___	
	___@___, ___@___, ___@___, ___@___, ___@___, ___@___	
	___@___, ___@___, ___@___, ___@___, ___@___, ___@___	
	___@___, ___@___, ___@___, ___@___, ___@___, ___@___	
	___@___, ___@___, ___@___, ___@___, ___@___, ___@___	
	___@___, ___@___, ___@___, ___@___, ___@___, ___@___	
	___@___, ___@___, ___@___, ___@___, ___@___, ___@___	
	___@___, ___@___, ___@___, ___@___, ___@___, ___@___	
	___@___, ___@___, ___@___, ___@___, ___@___, ___@___	
	___@___, ___@___, ___@___, ___@___, ___@___, ___@___	

<table>
<tr><td colspan="5" align="center">**Mechanical Theme**</td></tr>
<tr><td colspan="5" align="center">Mob. > Corr. > Fun. Stability > NM Efficiency > Musc. Endurance > Hypertrophy > Heavy Power > Max Power > A.M.S.</td></tr>
<tr><td colspan="5" align="center">**Metabolic Theme**
Met. Stim. > Aero. Elevation > Thresh. Development > Aero. Capacity > An. Expansion > Spec. Movements > Spec. Skills</td></tr>
</table>

Date	Warm Up		Cool Down		Movements/ Focus Area
	Exercise	*Duration*	*Exercise*	*Duration*	
___ / ___ / ___					

Activity	Rx (reps/dist. @ weight/time)	Rest
	____@____, ____@____, ____@____,	
	____@____, ____@____, ____@____	
	____@____, ____@____, ____@____,	
	____@____, ____@____, ____@____	
	____@____, ____@____, ____@____,	
	____@____, ____@____, ____@____	
	____@____, ____@____, ____@____,	
	____@____, ____@____, ____@____	
	____@____, ____@____, ____@____,	
	____@____, ____@____, ____@____	
	____@____, ____@____, ____@____,	
	____@____, ____@____, ____@____	
	____@____, ____@____, ____@____,	
	____@____, ____@____, ____@____	
	____@____, ____@____, ____@____,	
	____@____, ____@____, ____@____	
	____@____, ____@____, ____@____,	
	____@____, ____@____, ____@____	
	____@____, ____@____, ____@____,	
	____@____, ____@____, ____@____	

Mechanical Theme				
Mob. > Corr. > Fun. Stability > NM Efficiency > Musc. Endurance > Hypertrophy > Heavy Power > Max Power > A.M.S.				

Metabolic Theme				
Met. Stim. > Aero. Elevation > Thresh. Development > Aero. Capacity > An. Expansion > Spec. Movements > Spec. Skills				

Date	Warm Up		Cool Down		Movements/ Focus Area
	Exercise	*Duration*	*Exercise*	*Duration*	
__ / __ / __					

Activity	Rx (reps/dist. @ weight/time)	Rest
	___@___, ___@___, ___@___, ___@___, ___@___, ___@___	
	___@___, ___@___, ___@___, ___@___, ___@___, ___@___	
	___@___, ___@___, ___@___, ___@___, ___@___, ___@___	
	___@___, ___@___, ___@___, ___@___, ___@___, ___@___	
	___@___, ___@___, ___@___, ___@___, ___@___, ___@___	
	___@___, ___@___, ___@___, ___@___, ___@___, ___@___	
	___@___, ___@___, ___@___, ___@___, ___@___, ___@___	
	___@___, ___@___, ___@___, ___@___, ___@___, ___@___	
	___@___, ___@___, ___@___, ___@___, ___@___, ___@___	
	___@___, ___@___, ___@___, ___@___, ___@___, ___@___	
	___@___, ___@___, ___@___, ___@___, ___@___, ___@___	

Mechanical Theme
Mob. > Corr. > Fun. Stability > NM Efficiency > Musc. Endurance > Hypertrophy > Heavy Power > Max Power > A.M.S.

Metabolic Theme
Met. Stim. > Aero. Elevation > Thresh. Development > Aero. Capacity > An. Expansion > Spec. Movements > Spec. Skills

Date	Warm Up		Cool Down		Movements/ Focus Area
	Exercise	*Duration*	*Exercise*	*Duration*	
__/__/__					

Activity	Rx (reps/dist. @ weight/time)	Rest
	___@___ , ___@___ , ___@___ ,	
	___@___ , ___@___ , ___@___	
	___@___ , ___@___ , ___@___ ,	
	___@___ , ___@___ , ___@___	
	___@___ , ___@___ , ___@___ ,	
	___@___ , ___@___ , ___@___	
	___@___ , ___@___ , ___@___ ,	
	___@___ , ___@___ , ___@___	
	___@___ , ___@___ , ___@___ ,	
	___@___ , ___@___ , ___@___	
	___@___ , ___@___ , ___@___ ,	
	___@___ , ___@___ , ___@___	
	___@___ , ___@___ , ___@___ ,	
	___@___ , ___@___ , ___@___	
	___@___ , ___@___ , ___@___ ,	
	___@___ , ___@___ , ___@___	
	___@___ , ___@___ , ___@___ ,	
	___@___ , ___@___ , ___@___	
	___@___ , ___@___ , ___@___ ,	
	___@___ , ___@___ , ___@___	
	___@___ , ___@___ , ___@___ ,	
	___@___ , ___@___ , ___@___	

Mechanical Theme
Mob. > Corr. > Fun. Stability > NM Efficiency > Musc. Endurance > Hypertrophy > Heavy Power > Max Power > A.M.S.

Metabolic Theme
Met. Stim. > Aero. Elevation > Thresh. Development > Aero. Capacity > An. Expansion > Spec. Movements > Spec. Skills

Date	Warm Up		Cool Down		Movements/ Focus Area
	Exercise	*Duration*	*Exercise*	*Duration*	
___/___/___					

Activity	**Rx** (reps/dist. @ weight/time)	Rest
	____@____, ____@____, ____@____, ____@____, ____@____, ____@____	
	____@____, ____@____, ____@____, ____@____, ____@____, ____@____	
	____@____, ____@____, ____@____, ____@____, ____@____, ____@____	
	____@____, ____@____, ____@____, ____@____, ____@____, ____@____	
	____@____, ____@____, ____@____, ____@____, ____@____, ____@____	
	____@____, ____@____, ____@____, ____@____, ____@____, ____@____	
	____@____, ____@____, ____@____, ____@____, ____@____, ____@____	
	____@____, ____@____, ____@____, ____@____, ____@____, ____@____	
	____@____, ____@____, ____@____, ____@____, ____@____, ____@____	
	____@____, ____@____, ____@____, ____@____, ____@____, ____@____	

Mechanical Theme
Mob. > Corr. > Fun. Stability > NM Efficiency > Musc. Endurance > Hypertrophy > Heavy Power > Max Power > A.M.S.

Metabolic Theme
Met. Stim. > Aero. Elevation > Thresh. Development > Aero. Capacity > An. Expansion > Spec. Movements > Spec. Skills

Date	Warm Up		Cool Down		Movements/ Focus Area
	Exercise	*Duration*	*Exercise*	*Duration*	
___/___/___					

Activity	Rx (reps/dist. @ weight/time)	Rest
	___@___, ___@___, ___@___,	
	___@___, ___@___, ___@___	
	___@___, ___@___, ___@___,	
	___@___, ___@___, ___@___	
	___@___, ___@___, ___@___,	
	___@___, ___@___, ___@___	
	___@___, ___@___, ___@___,	
	___@___, ___@___, ___@___	
	___@___, ___@___, ___@___,	
	___@___, ___@___, ___@___	
	___@___, ___@___, ___@___,	
	___@___, ___@___, ___@___	
	___@___, ___@___, ___@___,	
	___@___, ___@___, ___@___	
	___@___, ___@___, ___@___,	
	___@___, ___@___, ___@___	
	___@___, ___@___, ___@___,	
	___@___, ___@___, ___@___	
	___@___, ___@___, ___@___,	
	___@___, ___@___, ___@___	
	___@___, ___@___, ___@___,	
	___@___, ___@___, ___@___	

Mechanical Theme

Mob. > Corr. > Fun. Stability > NM Efficiency > Musc. Endurance > Hypertrophy > Heavy Power > Max Power > A.M.S.

Metabolic Theme

Met. Stim. > Aero. Elevation > Thresh. Development > Aero. Capacity > An. Expansion > Spec. Movements > Spec. Skills

Date	Warm Up		Cool Down		Movements/ Focus Area
	Exercise	*Duration*	*Exercise*	*Duration*	
___ / ___ / ___					

Activity	Rx (reps/dist. @ weight/time)	Rest
	___@___, ___@___, ___@___, ___@___, ___@___, ___@___	
	___@___, ___@___, ___@___, ___@___, ___@___, ___@___	
	___@___, ___@___, ___@___, ___@___, ___@___, ___@___	
	___@___, ___@___, ___@___, ___@___, ___@___, ___@___	
	___@___, ___@___, ___@___, ___@___, ___@___, ___@___	
	___@___, ___@___, ___@___, ___@___, ___@___, ___@___	
	___@___, ___@___, ___@___, ___@___, ___@___, ___@___	
	___@___, ___@___, ___@___, ___@___, ___@___, ___@___	
	___@___, ___@___, ___@___, ___@___, ___@___, ___@___	
	___@___, ___@___, ___@___, ___@___, ___@___, ___@___	

Mechanical Theme

Mob. > Corr. > Fun. Stability > NM Efficiency > Musc. Endurance > Hypertrophy > Heavy Power > Max Power > A.M.S.

Metabolic Theme

Met. Stim. > Aero. Elevation > Thresh. Development > Aero. Capacity > An. Expansion > Spec. Movements > Spec. Skills

Date	Warm Up		Cool Down		Movements/ Focus Area
	Exercise	*Duration*	*Exercise*	*Duration*	
___/___/___					

Activity	Rx (reps/dist. @ weight/time)	Rest
	___@___, ___@___, ___@___,	
	___@___, ___@___, ___@___	
	___@___, ___@___, ___@___,	
	___@___, ___@___, ___@___	
	___@___, ___@___, ___@___,	
	___@___, ___@___, ___@___	
	___@___, ___@___, ___@___,	
	___@___, ___@___, ___@___	
	___@___, ___@___, ___@___,	
	___@___, ___@___, ___@___	
	___@___, ___@___, ___@___,	
	___@___, ___@___, ___@___	
	___@___, ___@___, ___@___,	
	___@___, ___@___, ___@___	
	___@___, ___@___, ___@___,	
	___@___, ___@___, ___@___	
	___@___, ___@___, ___@___,	
	___@___, ___@___, ___@___	
	___@___, ___@___, ___@___,	
	___@___, ___@___, ___@___	
	___@___, ___@___, ___@___,	
	___@___, ___@___, ___@___	

Mechanical Theme
Mob. > Corr. > Fun. Stability > NM Efficiency > Musc. Endurance > Hypertrophy > Heavy Power > Max Power > A.M.S.

Metabolic Theme
Met. Stim. > Aero. Elevation > Thresh. Development > Aero. Capacity > An. Expansion > Spec. Movements > Spec. Skills

Date	Warm Up		Cool Down		Movements/ Focus Area
	Exercise	*Duration*	*Exercise*	*Duration*	
__ / __ / __					

Activity	Rx (reps/dist. @ weight/time)	Rest
	___@___, ___@___, ___@___, ___@___, ___@___, ___@___	
	___@___, ___@___, ___@___, ___@___, ___@___, ___@___	
	___@___, ___@___, ___@___, ___@___, ___@___, ___@___	
	___@___, ___@___, ___@___, ___@___, ___@___, ___@___	
	___@___, ___@___, ___@___, ___@___, ___@___, ___@___	
	___@___, ___@___, ___@___, ___@___, ___@___, ___@___	
	___@___, ___@___, ___@___, ___@___, ___@___, ___@___	
	___@___, ___@___, ___@___, ___@___, ___@___, ___@___	
	___@___, ___@___, ___@___, ___@___, ___@___, ___@___	
	___@___, ___@___, ___@___, ___@___, ___@___, ___@___	

Mechanical Theme

Mob. > Corr. > Fun. Stability > NM Efficiency > Musc. Endurance > Hypertrophy > Heavy Power > Max Power > A.M.S.

Metabolic Theme

Met. Stim. > Aero. Elevation > Thresh. Development > Aero. Capacity > An. Expansion > Spec. Movements > Spec. Skills

Date	Warm Up		Cool Down		Movements/ Focus Area
	Exercise	*Duration*	*Exercise*	*Duration*	
__ / __ / __					

Activity	Rx (reps/dist. @ weight/time)	Rest
	___@___, ___@___, ___@___,	
	___@___, ___@___, ___@___	
	___@___, ___@___, ___@___,	
	___@___, ___@___, ___@___	
	___@___, ___@___, ___@___,	
	___@___, ___@___, ___@___	
	___@___, ___@___, ___@___,	
	___@___, ___@___, ___@___	
	___@___, ___@___, ___@___,	
	___@___, ___@___, ___@___	
	___@___, ___@___, ___@___,	
	___@___, ___@___, ___@___	
	___@___, ___@___, ___@___,	
	___@___, ___@___, ___@___	
	___@___, ___@___, ___@___,	
	___@___, ___@___, ___@___	
	___@___, ___@___, ___@___,	
	___@___, ___@___, ___@___	
	___@___, ___@___, ___@___,	
	___@___, ___@___, ___@___	
	___@___, ___@___, ___@___,	
	___@___, ___@___, ___@___	

Mechanical Theme
Mob. > Corr. > Fun. Stability > NM Efficiency > Musc. Endurance > Hypertrophy > Heavy Power > Max Power > A.M.S.

Metabolic Theme
Met. Stim. > Aero. Elevation > Thresh. Development > Aero. Capacity > An. Expansion > Spec. Movements > Spec. Skills

Date	Warm Up		Cool Down		Movements/ Focus Area
	Exercise	*Duration*	*Exercise*	*Duration*	
__/__/__					

Activity	Rx (reps/dist. @ weight/time)	Rest
	____@____, ____@____, ____@____, ____@____, ____@____, ____@____	
	____@____, ____@____, ____@____, ____@____, ____@____, ____@____	
	____@____, ____@____, ____@____, ____@____, ____@____, ____@____	
	____@____, ____@____, ____@____, ____@____, ____@____, ____@____	
	____@____, ____@____, ____@____, ____@____, ____@____, ____@____	
	____@____, ____@____, ____@____, ____@____, ____@____, ____@____	
	____@____, ____@____, ____@____, ____@____, ____@____, ____@____	
	____@____, ____@____, ____@____, ____@____, ____@____, ____@____	
	____@____, ____@____, ____@____, ____@____, ____@____, ____@____	
	____@____, ____@____, ____@____, ____@____, ____@____, ____@____	
	____@____, ____@____, ____@____, ____@____, ____@____, ____@____	

Mechanical Theme

Mob. > Corr. > Fun. Stability > NM Efficiency > Musc. Endurance > Hypertrophy > Heavy Power > Max Power > A.M.S.

Metabolic Theme

Met. Stim. > Aero. Elevation > Thresh. Development > Aero. Capacity > An. Expansion > Spec. Movements > Spec. Skills

Date	Warm Up		Cool Down		Movements/ Focus Area
	Exercise	*Duration*	*Exercise*	*Duration*	
___/___/___					

Activity	Rx (reps/dist. @ weight/time)	Rest
	____@____, ____@____, ____@____,	
	____@____, ____@____, ____@____	
	____@____, ____@____, ____@____,	
	____@____, ____@____, ____@____	
	____@____, ____@____, ____@____,	
	____@____, ____@____, ____@____	
	____@____, ____@____, ____@____,	
	____@____, ____@____, ____@____	
	____@____, ____@____, ____@____,	
	____@____, ____@____, ____@____	
	____@____, ____@____, ____@____,	
	____@____, ____@____, ____@____	
	____@____, ____@____, ____@____,	
	____@____, ____@____, ____@____	
	____@____, ____@____, ____@____,	
	____@____, ____@____, ____@____	
	____@____, ____@____, ____@____,	
	____@____, ____@____, ____@____	

Mechanical Theme
Mob. > Corr. > Fun. Stability > NM Efficiency > Musc. Endurance > Hypertrophy > Heavy Power > Max Power > A.M.S.

Metabolic Theme
Met. Stim. > Aero. Elevation > Thresh. Development > Aero. Capacity > An. Expansion > Spec. Movements > Spec. Skills

Date	Warm Up		Cool Down		Movements/ Focus Area
	Exercise	*Duration*	*Exercise*	*Duration*	
___/___/___					

Activity	**Rx** (reps/dist. @ weight/time)	Rest
	____@____, ____@____, ____@____, ____@____, ____@____, ____@____	
	____@____, ____@____, ____@____, ____@____, ____@____, ____@____	
	____@____, ____@____, ____@____, ____@____, ____@____, ____@____	
	____@____, ____@____, ____@____, ____@____, ____@____, ____@____	
	____@____, ____@____, ____@____, ____@____, ____@____, ____@____	
	____@____, ____@____, ____@____, ____@____, ____@____, ____@____	
	____@____, ____@____, ____@____, ____@____, ____@____, ____@____	
	____@____, ____@____, ____@____, ____@____, ____@____, ____@____	
	____@____, ____@____, ____@____, ____@____, ____@____, ____@____	
	____@____, ____@____, ____@____, ____@____, ____@____, ____@____	

Mechanical Theme
Mob. > Corr. > Fun. Stability > NM Efficiency > Musc. Endurance > Hypertrophy > Heavy Power > Max Power > A.M.S.

Metabolic Theme
Met. Stim. > Aero. Elevation > Thresh. Development > Aero. Capacity > An. Expansion > Spec. Movements > Spec. Skills

Date	Warm Up		Cool Down		Movements/ Focus Area
	Exercise	*Duration*	*Exercise*	*Duration*	
__ / __ / __					

Activity	Rx (reps/dist. @ weight/time)	Rest
	____@____, ____@____, ____@____,	
	____@____, ____@____, ____@____	
	____@____, ____@____, ____@____,	
	____@____, ____@____, ____@____	
	____@____, ____@____, ____@____,	
	____@____, ____@____, ____@____	
	____@____, ____@____, ____@____,	
	____@____, ____@____, ____@____	
	____@____, ____@____, ____@____,	
	____@____, ____@____, ____@____	
	____@____, ____@____, ____@____,	
	____@____, ____@____, ____@____	
	____@____, ____@____, ____@____,	
	____@____, ____@____, ____@____	
	____@____, ____@____, ____@____,	
	____@____, ____@____, ____@____	
	____@____, ____@____, ____@____,	
	____@____, ____@____, ____@____	
	____@____, ____@____, ____@____,	
	____@____, ____@____, ____@____	

Mechanical Theme
Mob. > Corr. > Fun. Stability > NM Efficiency > Musc. Endurance > Hypertrophy > Heavy Power > Max Power > A.M.S.

Metabolic Theme
Met. Stim. > Aero. Elevation > Thresh. Development > Aero. Capacity > An. Expansion > Spec. Movements > Spec. Skills

Date	Warm Up		Cool Down		Movements/ Focus Area
	Exercise	*Duration*	*Exercise*	*Duration*	
___/___/___					

Activity	Rx (reps/dist. @ weight/time)	Rest
	_@____, ____@____, ____@____, _@____, ____@____, ____@____	
	_@____, ____@____, ____@____, _@____, ____@____, ____@____	
	_@____, ____@____, ____@____, _@____, ____@____, ____@____	
	_@____, ____@____, ____@____, _@____, ____@____, ____@____	
	_@____, ____@____, ____@____, _@____, ____@____, ____@____	
	_@____, ____@____, ____@____, _@____, ____@____, ____@____	
	_@____, ____@____, ____@____, _@____, ____@____, ____@____	
	_@____, ____@____, ____@____, _@____, ____@____, ____@____	
	_@____, ____@____, ____@____, _@____, ____@____, ____@____	
	_@____, ____@____, ____@____, _@____, ____@____, ____@____	

Mechanical Theme
Mob. > Corr. > Fun. Stability > NM Efficiency > Musc. Endurance > Hypertrophy > Heavy Power > Max Power > A.M.S.

Metabolic Theme
Met. Stim. > Aero. Elevation > Thresh. Development > Aero. Capacity > An. Expansion > Spec. Movements > Spec. Skills

Date	Warm Up		Cool Down		Movements/ Focus Area
	Exercise	*Duration*	*Exercise*	*Duration*	
___/___/___					

Activity	Rx (reps/dist. @ weight/time)	Rest
	____@____, ____@____, ____@____,	
	____@____, ____@____, ____@____	
	____@____, ____@____, ____@____,	
	____@____, ____@____, ____@____	
	____@____, ____@____, ____@____,	
	____@____, ____@____, ____@____	
	____@____, ____@____, ____@____,	
	____@____, ____@____, ____@____	
	____@____, ____@____, ____@____,	
	____@____, ____@____, ____@____	
	____@____, ____@____, ____@____,	
	____@____, ____@____, ____@____	
	____@____, ____@____, ____@____,	
	____@____, ____@____, ____@____	
	____@____, ____@____, ____@____,	
	____@____, ____@____, ____@____	
	____@____, ____@____, ____@____,	
	____@____, ____@____, ____@____	
	____@____, ____@____, ____@____,	
	____@____, ____@____, ____@____	

Mechanical Theme
Mob. > Corr. > Fun. Stability > NM Efficiency > Musc. Endurance > Hypertrophy > Heavy Power > Max Power > A.M.S.

Metabolic Theme
Met. Stim. > Aero. Elevation > Thresh. Development > Aero. Capacity > An. Expansion > Spec. Movements > Spec. Skills

Date	Warm Up		Cool Down		Movements/ Focus Area
	Exercise	*Duration*	*Exercise*	*Duration*	
___/___/___					

Activity	Rx (reps/dist. @ weight/time)	Rest
	____@____, ____@____, ____@____, ____@____, ____@____, ____@____	
	____@____, ____@____, ____@____, ____@____, ____@____, ____@____	
	____@____, ____@____, ____@____, ____@____, ____@____, ____@____	
	____@____, ____@____, ____@____, ____@____, ____@____, ____@____	
	____@____, ____@____, ____@____, ____@____, ____@____, ____@____	
	____@____, ____@____, ____@____, ____@____, ____@____, ____@____	
	____@____, ____@____, ____@____, ____@____, ____@____, ____@____	
	____@____, ____@____, ____@____, ____@____, ____@____, ____@____	
	____@____, ____@____, ____@____, ____@____, ____@____, ____@____	
	____@____, ____@____, ____@____, ____@____, ____@____, ____@____	

Mechanical Theme
Mob. > Corr. > Fun. Stability > NM Efficiency > Musc. Endurance > Hypertrophy > Heavy Power > Max Power > A.M.S.

Metabolic Theme
Met. Stim. > Aero. Elevation > Thresh. Development > Aero. Capacity > An. Expansion > Spec. Movements > Spec. Skills

Date	Warm Up		Cool Down		Movements/ Focus Area
	Exercise	*Duration*	*Exercise*	*Duration*	
___ / ___ / ___					

Activity	Rx (reps/dist. @ weight/time)	Rest
	____ @____ , ____ @____ , ____ @____ ,	
	____ @____ , ____ @____ , ____ @____	
	____ @____ , ____ @____ , ____ @____ ,	
	____ @____ , ____ @____ , ____ @____	
	____ @____ , ____ @____ , ____ @____ ,	
	____ @____ , ____ @____ , ____ @____	
	____ @____ , ____ @____ , ____ @____ ,	
	____ @____ , ____ @____ , ____ @____	
	____ @____ , ____ @____ , ____ @____ ,	
	____ @____ , ____ @____ , ____ @____	
	____ @____ , ____ @____ , ____ @____ ,	
	____ @____ , ____ @____ , ____ @____	
	____ @____ , ____ @____ , ____ @____ ,	
	____ @____ , ____ @____ , ____ @____	
	____ @____ , ____ @____ , ____ @____ ,	
	____ @____ , ____ @____ , ____ @____	
	____ @____ , ____ @____ , ____ @____ ,	
	____ @____ , ____ @____ , ____ @____	
	____ @____ , ____ @____ , ____ @____ ,	
	____ @____ , ____ @____ , ____ @____	

Mechanical Theme
Mob. > Corr. > Fun. Stability > NM Efficiency > Musc. Endurance > Hypertrophy > Heavy Power > Max Power > A.M.S.

Metabolic Theme
Met. Stim. > Aero. Elevation > Thresh. Development > Aero. Capacity > An. Expansion > Spec. Movements > Spec. Skills

Date	Warm Up		Cool Down		Movements/ Focus Area
	Exercise	*Duration*	*Exercise*	*Duration*	
___ / ___ / ___					

Activity	Rx (reps/dist. @ weight/time)	Rest
	@____, ____ @____, ____ @____, @____, ____ @____, ____ @____	
	@____, ____ @____, ____ @____, @____, ____ @____, ____ @____	
	@____, ____ @____, ____ @____, @____, ____ @____, ____ @____	
	@____, ____ @____, ____ @____, @____, ____ @____, ____ @____	
	@____, ____ @____, ____ @____, @____, ____ @____, ____ @____	
	@____, ____ @____, ____ @____, @____, ____ @____, ____ @____	
	@____, ____ @____, ____ @____, @____, ____ @____, ____ @____	
	@____, ____ @____, ____ @____, @____, ____ @____, ____ @____	
	@____, ____ @____, ____ @____, @____, ____ @____, ____ @____	
	@____, ____ @____, ____ @____	

Mechanical Theme

Mob. > Corr. > Fun. Stability > NM Efficiency > Musc. Endurance > Hypertrophy > Heavy Power > Max Power > A.M.S.

Metabolic Theme

Met. Stim. > Aero. Elevation > Thresh. Development > Aero. Capacity > An. Expansion > Spec. Movements > Spec. Skills

Date	Warm Up		Cool Down		Movements/ Focus Area
	Exercise	*Duration*	*Exercise*	*Duration*	
__/__/__					

Activity	Rx (reps/dist. @ weight/time)	Rest
	__@__, __@__, __@__,	
	__@__, __@__, __@__	
	__@__, __@__, __@__,	
	__@__, __@__, __@__	
	__@__, __@__, __@__,	
	__@__, __@__, __@__	
	__@__, __@__, __@__,	
	__@__, __@__, __@__	
	__@__, __@__, __@__,	
	__@__, __@__, __@__	
	__@__, __@__, __@__,	
	__@__, __@__, __@__	
	__@__, __@__, __@__,	
	__@__, __@__, __@__	
	__@__, __@__, __@__,	
	__@__, __@__, __@__	
	__@__, __@__, __@__,	
	__@__, __@__, __@__	
	__@__, __@__, __@__,	
	__@__, __@__, __@__	

Mechanical Theme

Mob. > Corr. > Fun. Stability > NM Efficiency > Musc. Endurance > Hypertrophy > Heavy Power > Max Power > A.M.S.

Metabolic Theme

Met. Stim. > Aero. Elevation > Thresh. Development > Aero. Capacity > An. Expansion > Spec. Movements > Spec. Skills

Date	Warm Up		Cool Down		Movements/ Focus Area
	Exercise	*Duration*	*Exercise*	*Duration*	
___/___/___					

Activity	Rx (reps/dist. @ weight/time)	Rest
	___@___, ___@___, ___@___, ___@___, ___@___, ___@___	
	___@___, ___@___, ___@___, ___@___, ___@___, ___@___	
	___@___, ___@___, ___@___, ___@___, ___@___, ___@___	
	___@___, ___@___, ___@___, ___@___, ___@___, ___@___	
	___@___, ___@___, ___@___, ___@___, ___@___, ___@___	
	___@___, ___@___, ___@___, ___@___, ___@___, ___@___	
	___@___, ___@___, ___@___, ___@___, ___@___, ___@___	
	___@___, ___@___, ___@___, ___@___, ___@___, ___@___	
	___@___, ___@___, ___@___, ___@___, ___@___, ___@___	
	___@___, ___@___, ___@___, ___@___, ___@___, ___@___	

Mechanical Theme
Mob. > Corr. > Fun. Stability > NM Efficiency > Musc. Endurance > Hypertrophy > Heavy Power > Max Power > A.M.S.

Metabolic Theme
Met. Stim. > Aero. Elevation > Thresh. Development > Aero. Capacity > An. Expansion > Spec. Movements > Spec. Skills

Date	Warm Up		Cool Down		Movements/ Focus Area
	Exercise	*Duration*	*Exercise*	*Duration*	
__/__/__					

Activity	Rx (reps/dist. @ weight/time)	Rest
	___@___, ___@___, ___@___,	
	___@___, ___@___, ___@___	
	___@___, ___@___, ___@___,	
	___@___, ___@___, ___@___	
	___@___, ___@___, ___@___,	
	___@___, ___@___, ___@___	
	___@___, ___@___, ___@___,	
	___@___, ___@___, ___@___	
	___@___, ___@___, ___@___,	
	___@___, ___@___, ___@___	
	___@___, ___@___, ___@___,	
	___@___, ___@___, ___@___	
	___@___, ___@___, ___@___,	
	___@___, ___@___, ___@___	
	___@___, ___@___, ___@___,	
	___@___, ___@___, ___@___	
	___@___, ___@___, ___@___,	
	___@___, ___@___, ___@___	
	___@___, ___@___, ___@___,	
	___@___, ___@___, ___@___	
	___@___, ___@___, ___@___,	
	___@___, ___@___, ___@___	

Mechanical Theme
Mob. > Corr. > Fun. Stability > NM Efficiency > Musc. Endurance > Hypertrophy > Heavy Power > Max Power > A.M.S.

Metabolic Theme
Met. Stim. > Aero. Elevation > Thresh. Development > Aero. Capacity > An. Expansion > Spec. Movements > Spec. Skills

Date	Warm Up		Cool Down		Movements/ Focus Area
	Exercise	*Duration*	*Exercise*	*Duration*	
___ / ___ / ___					

Activity	Rx (reps/dist. @ weight/time)	Rest
	____@____, ____@____, ____@____, ____@____, ____@____, ____@____	
	____@____, ____@____, ____@____, ____@____, ____@____, ____@____	
	____@____, ____@____, ____@____, ____@____, ____@____, ____@____	
	____@____, ____@____, ____@____, ____@____, ____@____, ____@____	
	____@____, ____@____, ____@____, ____@____, ____@____, ____@____	
	____@____, ____@____, ____@____, ____@____, ____@____, ____@____	
	____@____, ____@____, ____@____, ____@____, ____@____, ____@____	
	____@____, ____@____, ____@____, ____@____, ____@____, ____@____	
	____@____, ____@____, ____@____, ____@____, ____@____, ____@____	
	____@____, ____@____, ____@____, ____@____, ____@____, ____@____	

Mechanical Theme
Mob. > Corr. > Fun. Stability > NM Efficiency > Musc. Endurance > Hypertrophy > Heavy Power > Max Power > A.M.S.

Metabolic Theme
Met. Stim. > Aero. Elevation > Thresh. Development > Aero. Capacity > An. Expansion > Spec. Movements > Spec. Skills

Date	Warm Up		Cool Down		Movements/ Focus Area
	Exercise	*Duration*	*Exercise*	*Duration*	
___/___/___					

Activity	Rx (reps/dist. @ weight/time)			Rest
	___@___,	___@___,	___@___,	
	___@___,	___@___,	___@___	
	___@___,	___@___,	___@___,	
	___@___,	___@___,	___@___	
	___@___,	___@___,	___@___,	
	___@___,	___@___,	___@___	
	___@___,	___@___,	___@___,	
	___@___,	___@___,	___@___	
	___@___,	___@___,	___@___,	
	___@___,	___@___,	___@___	
	___@___,	___@___,	___@___,	
	___@___,	___@___,	___@___	
	___@___,	___@___,	___@___,	
	___@___,	___@___,	___@___	
	___@___,	___@___,	___@___,	
	___@___,	___@___,	___@___	
	___@___,	___@___,	___@___,	
	___@___,	___@___,	___@___	
	___@___,	___@___,	___@___,	
	___@___,	___@___,	___@___	
	___@___,	___@___,	___@___,	
	___@___,	___@___,	___@___	

Mechanical Theme
Mob. > Corr. > Fun. Stability > NM Efficiency > Musc. Endurance > Hypertrophy > Heavy Power > Max Power > A.M.S.

Metabolic Theme
Met. Stim. > Aero. Elevation > Thresh. Development > Aero. Capacity > An. Expansion > Spec. Movements > Spec. Skills

Date	Warm Up		Cool Down		Movements/ Focus Area
	Exercise	*Duration*	*Exercise*	*Duration*	
___/___/___					

Activity	Rx (reps/dist. @ weight/time)	Rest
	____@____, ____@____, ____@____, ____@____, ____@____, ____@____	
	____@____, ____@____, ____@____, ____@____, ____@____, ____@____	
	____@____, ____@____, ____@____, ____@____, ____@____, ____@____	
	____@____, ____@____, ____@____, ____@____, ____@____, ____@____	
	____@____, ____@____, ____@____, ____@____, ____@____, ____@____	
	____@____, ____@____, ____@____, ____@____, ____@____, ____@____	
	____@____, ____@____, ____@____, ____@____, ____@____, ____@____	
	____@____, ____@____, ____@____, ____@____, ____@____, ____@____	
	____@____, ____@____, ____@____, ____@____, ____@____, ____@____	
	____@____, ____@____, ____@____, ____@____, ____@____, ____@____	

Mechanical Theme
Mob. > Corr. > Fun. Stability > NM Efficiency > Musc. Endurance > Hypertrophy > Heavy Power > Max Power > A.M.S.

Metabolic Theme
Met. Stim. > Aero. Elevation > Thresh. Development > Aero. Capacity > An. Expansion > Spec. Movements > Spec. Skills

Date	Warm Up		Cool Down		Movements/ Focus Area
	Exercise	*Duration*	*Exercise*	*Duration*	
___ / ___ / ___					

Activity	Rx (reps/dist. @ weight/time)	Rest
	_____ @_____ , _____ @_____ , _____ @_____ ,	
	_____ @_____ , _____ @_____ , _____ @_____	
	_____ @_____ , _____ @_____ , _____ @_____ ,	
	_____ @_____ , _____ @_____ , _____ @_____	
	_____ @_____ , _____ @_____ , _____ @_____ ,	
	_____ @_____ , _____ @_____ , _____ @_____	
	_____ @_____ , _____ @_____ , _____ @_____ ,	
	_____ @_____ , _____ @_____ , _____ @_____	
	_____ @_____ , _____ @_____ , _____ @_____ ,	
	_____ @_____ , _____ @_____ , _____ @_____	
	_____ @_____ , _____ @_____ , _____ @_____ ,	
	_____ @_____ , _____ @_____ , _____ @_____	
	_____ @_____ , _____ @_____ , _____ @_____ ,	
	_____ @_____ , _____ @_____ , _____ @_____	
	_____ @_____ , _____ @_____ , _____ @_____ ,	
	_____ @_____ , _____ @_____ , _____ @_____	
	_____ @_____ , _____ @_____ , _____ @_____ ,	
	_____ @_____ , _____ @_____ , _____ @_____	
	_____ @_____ , _____ @_____ , _____ @_____ ,	
	_____ @_____ , _____ @_____ , _____ @_____	
	_____ @_____ , _____ @_____ , _____ @_____ ,	
	_____ @_____ , _____ @_____ , _____ @_____	

Mechanical Theme

Mob. > Corr. > Fun. Stability > NM Efficiency > Musc. Endurance > Hypertrophy > Heavy Power > Max Power > A.M.S.

Metabolic Theme

Met. Stim. > Aero. Elevation > Thresh. Development > Aero. Capacity > An. Expansion > Spec. Movements > Spec. Skills

Date	Warm Up		Cool Down		Movements/ Focus Area
	Exercise	*Duration*	*Exercise*	*Duration*	
___/___/___					

Activity	**Rx** (reps/dist. @ weight/time)	Rest
	___@___, ___@___, ___@___,	
	___@___, ___@___, ___@___	
	___@___, ___@___, ___@___,	
	___@___, ___@___, ___@___	
	___@___, ___@___, ___@___,	
	___@___, ___@___, ___@___	
	___@___, ___@___, ___@___,	
	___@___, ___@___, ___@___	
	___@___, ___@___, ___@___,	
	___@___, ___@___, ___@___	
	___@___, ___@___, ___@___,	
	___@___, ___@___, ___@___	
	___@___, ___@___, ___@___,	
	___@___, ___@___, ___@___	
	___@___, ___@___, ___@___,	
	___@___, ___@___, ___@___	
	___@___, ___@___, ___@___,	
	___@___, ___@___, ___@___	
	___@___, ___@___, ___@___,	
	___@___, ___@___, ___@___	

Mechanical Theme
Mob. > Corr. > Fun. Stability > NM Efficiency > Musc. Endurance > Hypertrophy > Heavy Power > Max Power > A.M.S.

Metabolic Theme
Met. Stim. > Aero. Elevation > Thresh. Development > Aero. Capacity > An. Expansion > Spec. Movements > Spec. Skills

Date	Warm Up		Cool Down		Movements/ Focus Area
	Exercise	*Duration*	*Exercise*	*Duration*	
___ / ___ / ___					

Activity	Rx (reps/dist. @ weight/time)	Rest
	_____@_____, _____@_____, _____@_____,	
	_____@_____, _____@_____, _____@_____	
	_____@_____, _____@_____, _____@_____,	
	_____@_____, _____@_____, _____@_____	
	_____@_____, _____@_____, _____@_____,	
	_____@_____, _____@_____, _____@_____	
	_____@_____, _____@_____, _____@_____,	
	_____@_____, _____@_____, _____@_____	
	_____@_____, _____@_____, _____@_____,	
	_____@_____, _____@_____, _____@_____	
	_____@_____, _____@_____, _____@_____,	
	_____@_____, _____@_____, _____@_____	
	_____@_____, _____@_____, _____@_____,	
	_____@_____, _____@_____, _____@_____	
	_____@_____, _____@_____, _____@_____,	
	_____@_____, _____@_____, _____@_____	
	_____@_____, _____@_____, _____@_____,	
	_____@_____, _____@_____, _____@_____	
	_____@_____, _____@_____, _____@_____,	
	_____@_____, _____@_____, _____@_____	

Mechanical Theme
Mob. > Corr. > Fun. Stability > NM Efficiency > Musc. Endurance > Hypertrophy > Heavy Power > Max Power > A.M.S.

Metabolic Theme
Met. Stim. > Aero. Elevation > Thresh. Development > Aero. Capacity > An. Expansion > Spec. Movements > Spec. Skills

Date	Warm Up		Cool Down		Movements/ Focus Area
	Exercise	*Duration*	*Exercise*	*Duration*	
___/___/___					

Activity	Rx (reps/dist. @ weight/time)	Rest
	____@____, ____@____, ____@____, ____@____, ____@____, ____@____	
	____@____, ____@____, ____@____, ____@____, ____@____, ____@____	
	____@____, ____@____, ____@____, ____@____, ____@____, ____@____	
	____@____, ____@____, ____@____, ____@____, ____@____, ____@____	
	____@____, ____@____, ____@____, ____@____, ____@____, ____@____	
	____@____, ____@____, ____@____, ____@____, ____@____, ____@____	
	____@____, ____@____, ____@____, ____@____, ____@____, ____@____	
	____@____, ____@____, ____@____, ____@____, ____@____, ____@____	
	____@____, ____@____, ____@____, ____@____, ____@____, ____@____	
	____@____, ____@____, ____@____, ____@____, ____@____, ____@____	

Mechanical Theme

Mob. > Corr. > Fun. Stability > NM Efficiency > Musc. Endurance > Hypertrophy > Heavy Power > Max Power > A.M.S.

Metabolic Theme

Met. Stim. > Aero. Elevation > Thresh. Development > Aero. Capacity > An. Expansion > Spec. Movements > Spec. Skills

Date	Warm Up		Cool Down		Movements/ Focus Area
	Exercise	*Duration*	*Exercise*	*Duration*	
___/___/___					

Activity	Rx (reps/dist. @ weight/time)	Rest
	____@____, ____@____, ____@____,	
	____@____, ____@____, ____@	
	____@____, ____@____, ____@____,	
	____@____, ____@____, ____@	
	____@____, ____@____, ____@____,	
	____@____, ____@____, ____@	
	____@____, ____@____, ____@____,	
	____@____, ____@____, ____@	
	____@____, ____@____, ____@____,	
	____@____, ____@____, ____@	
	____@____, ____@____, ____@____,	
	____@____, ____@____, ____@	
	____@____, ____@____, ____@____,	
	____@____, ____@____, ____@	
	____@____, ____@____, ____@____,	
	____@____, ____@____, ____@	
	____@____, ____@____, ____@____,	
	____@____, ____@____, ____@	
	____@____, ____@____, ____@____,	
	____@____, ____@____, ____@	

<table>
<tr><td colspan="5">Mechanical Theme
Mob. > Corr. > Fun. Stability > NM Efficiency > Musc. Endurance > Hypertrophy > Heavy Power > Max Power > A.M.S.</td></tr>
</table>

<table>
<tr><td>Metabolic Theme
Met. Stim. > Aero. Elevation > Thresh. Development > Aero. Capacity > An. Expansion > Spec. Movements > Spec. Skills</td></tr>
</table>

Date	Warm Up		Cool Down		Movements/ Focus Area
	Exercise	*Duration*	*Exercise*	*Duration*	
___/___/___					

Activity	**Rx** (reps/dist. @ weight/time)	Rest
	____@____, ____@____, ____@____, ____@____, ____@____, ____@____	
	____@____, ____@____, ____@____, ____@____, ____@____, ____@____	
	____@____, ____@____, ____@____, ____@____, ____@____, ____@____	
	____@____, ____@____, ____@____, ____@____, ____@____, ____@____	
	____@____, ____@____, ____@____, ____@____, ____@____, ____@____	
	____@____, ____@____, ____@____, ____@____, ____@____, ____@____	
	____@____, ____@____, ____@____, ____@____, ____@____, ____@____	
	____@____, ____@____, ____@____, ____@____, ____@____, ____@____	
	____@____, ____@____, ____@____, ____@____, ____@____, ____@____	
	____@____, ____@____, ____@____, ____@____, ____@____, ____@____	

Mechanical Theme
Mob. > Corr. > Fun. Stability > NM Efficiency > Musc. Endurance > Hypertrophy > Heavy Power > Max Power > A.M.S.

Metabolic Theme
Met. Stim. > Aero. Elevation > Thresh. Development > Aero. Capacity > An. Expansion > Spec. Movements > Spec. Skills

Date	Warm Up		Cool Down		Movements/ Focus Area
	Exercise	*Duration*	*Exercise*	*Duration*	
___/___/___					

Activity	Rx (reps/dist. @ weight/time)	Rest
	____@____, ____@____, ____@____,	
	____@____, ____@____, ____@____	
	____@____, ____@____, ____@____,	
	____@____, ____@____, ____@____	
	____@____, ____@____, ____@____,	
	____@____, ____@____, ____@____	
	____@____, ____@____, ____@____,	
	____@____, ____@____, ____@____	
	____@____, ____@____, ____@____,	
	____@____, ____@____, ____@____	
	____@____, ____@____, ____@____,	
	____@____, ____@____, ____@____	
	____@____, ____@____, ____@____,	
	____@____, ____@____, ____@____	
	____@____, ____@____, ____@____,	
	____@____, ____@____, ____@____	
	____@____, ____@____, ____@____,	
	____@____, ____@____, ____@____	
	____@____, ____@____, ____@____,	
	____@____, ____@____, ____@____	
	____@____, ____@____, ____@____,	
	____@____, ____@____, ____@____	

Mechanical Theme
Mob. > Corr. > Fun. Stability > NM Efficiency > Musc. Endurance > Hypertrophy > Heavy Power > Max Power > A.M.S.

Metabolic Theme
Met. Stim. > Aero. Elevation > Thresh. Development > Aero. Capacity > An. Expansion > Spec. Movements > Spec. Skills

Date	Warm Up		Cool Down		Movements/ Focus Area
	Exercise	*Duration*	*Exercise*	*Duration*	
___/___/___					

Activity	Rx (reps/dist. @ weight/time)	Rest
	____@____, ____@____, ____@____, ____@____, ____@____, ____@____	
	____@____, ____@____, ____@____, ____@____, ____@____, ____@____	
	____@____, ____@____, ____@____, ____@____, ____@____, ____@____	
	____@____, ____@____, ____@____, ____@____, ____@____, ____@____	
	____@____, ____@____, ____@____, ____@____, ____@____, ____@____	
	____@____, ____@____, ____@____, ____@____, ____@____, ____@____	
	____@____, ____@____, ____@____, ____@____, ____@____, ____@____	
	____@____, ____@____, ____@____, ____@____, ____@____, ____@____	
	____@____, ____@____, ____@____, ____@____, ____@____, ____@____	
	____@____, ____@____, ____@____, ____@____, ____@____, ____@____	

Mechanical Theme
Mob. > Corr. > Fun. Stability > NM Efficiency > Musc. Endurance > Hypertrophy > Heavy Power > Max Power > A.M.S.

Metabolic Theme
Met. Stim. > Aero. Elevation > Thresh. Development > Aero. Capacity > An. Expansion > Spec. Movements > Spec. Skills

Date	Warm Up		Cool Down		Movements/ Focus Area
	Exercise	*Duration*	*Exercise*	*Duration*	
___ / ___ / ___					

Activity	**Rx** (reps/dist. @ weight/time)	Rest
	____@____, ____@____, ____@____,	
	____@____, ____@____, ____@____	
	____@____, ____@____, ____@____,	
	____@____, ____@____, ____@____	
	____@____, ____@____, ____@____,	
	____@____, ____@____, ____@____	
	____@____, ____@____, ____@____,	
	____@____, ____@____, ____@____	
	____@____, ____@____, ____@____,	
	____@____, ____@____, ____@____	
	____@____, ____@____, ____@____,	
	____@____, ____@____, ____@____	
	____@____, ____@____, ____@____,	
	____@____, ____@____, ____@____	
	____@____, ____@____, ____@____,	
	____@____, ____@____, ____@____	
	____@____, ____@____, ____@____,	
	____@____, ____@____, ____@____	
	____@____, ____@____, ____@____,	
	____@____, ____@____, ____@____	

Mechanical Theme
Mob. > Corr. > Fun. Stability > NM Efficiency > Musc. Endurance > Hypertrophy > Heavy Power > Max Power > A.M.S.

Metabolic Theme
Met. Stim. > Aero. Elevation > Thresh. Development > Aero. Capacity > An. Expansion > Spec. Movements > Spec. Skills

Date	Warm Up		Cool Down		Movements/ Focus Area
	Exercise	*Duration*	*Exercise*	*Duration*	
___/___/___					

Activity	Rx (reps/dist. @ weight/time)	Rest
	____@____, ____@____, ____@____, ____@____, ____@____, ____@____	
	____@____, ____@____, ____@____, ____@____, ____@____, ____@____	
	____@____, ____@____, ____@____, ____@____, ____@____, ____@____	
	____@____, ____@____, ____@____, ____@____, ____@____, ____@____	
	____@____, ____@____, ____@____, ____@____, ____@____, ____@____	
	____@____, ____@____, ____@____, ____@____, ____@____, ____@____	
	____@____, ____@____, ____@____, ____@____, ____@____, ____@____	
	____@____, ____@____, ____@____, ____@____, ____@____, ____@____	
	____@____, ____@____, ____@____, ____@____, ____@____, ____@____	
	____@____, ____@____, ____@____, ____@____, ____@____, ____@____	
	____@____, ____@____, ____@____, ____@____, ____@____, ____@____	

Mechanical Theme
Mob. > Corr. > Fun. Stability > NM Efficiency > Musc. Endurance > Hypertrophy > Heavy Power > Max Power > A.M.S.

Metabolic Theme
Met. Stim. > Aero. Elevation > Thresh. Development > Aero. Capacity > An. Expansion > Spec. Movements > Spec. Skills

Date	Warm Up		Cool Down		Movements/ Focus Area
	Exercise	_Duration_	_Exercise_	_Duration_	
___/___/___					

Activity	Rx (reps/dist. @ weight/time)	Rest
	____@____, ____@____, ____@____,	
	@____, @____, @____	
	____@____, ____@____, ____@____,	
	@____, @____, @____	
	____@____, ____@____, ____@____,	
	@____, @____, @____	
	____@____, ____@____, ____@____,	
	@____, @____, @____	
	____@____, ____@____, ____@____,	
	@____, @____, @____	
	____@____, ____@____, ____@____,	
	@____, @____, @____	
	____@____, ____@____, ____@____,	
	@____, @____, @____	
	____@____, ____@____, ____@____,	
	@____, @____, @____	
	____@____, ____@____, ____@____,	
	@____, @____, @____	

Mechanical Theme
Mob. > Corr. > Fun. Stability > NM Efficiency > Musc. Endurance > Hypertrophy > Heavy Power > Max Power > A.M.S.

Metabolic Theme
Met. Stim. > Aero. Elevation > Thresh. Development > Aero. Capacity > An. Expansion > Spec. Movements > Spec. Skills

Date	Warm Up		Cool Down		Movements/ Focus Area
	Exercise	*Duration*	*Exercise*	*Duration*	
___/___/___					

Activity	Rx (reps/dist. @ weight/time)	Rest
	___@___, ___@___, ___@___, ___@___, ___@___, ___@___	
	___@___, ___@___, ___@___, ___@___, ___@___, ___@___	
	___@___, ___@___, ___@___, ___@___, ___@___, ___@___	
	___@___, ___@___, ___@___, ___@___, ___@___, ___@___	
	___@___, ___@___, ___@___, ___@___, ___@___, ___@___	
	___@___, ___@___, ___@___, ___@___, ___@___, ___@___	
	___@___, ___@___, ___@___, ___@___, ___@___, ___@___	
	___@___, ___@___, ___@___, ___@___, ___@___, ___@___	
	___@___, ___@___, ___@___, ___@___, ___@___, ___@___	
	___@___, ___@___, ___@___, ___@___, ___@___, ___@___	

Mechanical Theme
Mob. > Corr. > Fun. Stability > NM Efficiency > Musc. Endurance > Hypertrophy > Heavy Power > Max Power > A.M.S.

Metabolic Theme
Met. Stim. > Aero. Elevation > Thresh. Development > Aero. Capacity > An. Expansion > Spec. Movements > Spec. Skills

Date	Warm Up		Cool Down		Movements/ Focus Area
	Exercise	*Duration*	*Exercise*	*Duration*	
___ / ___ / ___					

Activity	**Rx** (reps/dist. @ weight/time)	Rest
	___@___ , ___@___ , ___@___ ,	
	___@___ , ___@___ , ___@___	
	___@___ , ___@___ , ___@___ ,	
	___@___ , ___@___ , ___@___	
	___@___ , ___@___ , ___@___ ,	
	___@___ , ___@___ , ___@___	
	___@___ , ___@___ , ___@___ ,	
	___@___ , ___@___ , ___@___	
	___@___ , ___@___ , ___@___ ,	
	___@___ , ___@___ , ___@___	
	___@___ , ___@___ , ___@___ ,	
	___@___ , ___@___ , ___@___	
	___@___ , ___@___ , ___@___ ,	
	___@___ , ___@___ , ___@___	
	___@___ , ___@___ , ___@___ ,	
	___@___ , ___@___ , ___@___	
	___@___ , ___@___ , ___@___ ,	
	___@___ , ___@___ , ___@___	
	___@___ , ___@___ , ___@___ ,	
	___@___ , ___@___ , ___@___	
	___@___ , ___@___ , ___@___ ,	
	___@___ , ___@___ , ___@___	

Mechanical Theme
Mob. > Corr. > Fun. Stability > NM Efficiency > Musc. Endurance > Hypertrophy > Heavy Power > Max Power > A.M.S.

Metabolic Theme
Met. Stim. > Aero. Elevation > Thresh. Development > Aero. Capacity > An. Expansion > Spec. Movements > Spec. Skills

Date	Warm Up		Cool Down		Movements/ Focus Area
	Exercise	*Duration*	*Exercise*	*Duration*	
___ / ___ / ___					

Activity	Rx (reps/dist. @ weight/time)	Rest
	____@____, ____@____, ____@____, ____@____, ____@____, ____@____	
	____@____, ____@____, ____@____, ____@____, ____@____, ____@____	
	____@____, ____@____, ____@____, ____@____, ____@____, ____@____	
	____@____, ____@____, ____@____, ____@____, ____@____, ____@____	
	____@____, ____@____, ____@____, ____@____, ____@____, ____@____	
	____@____, ____@____, ____@____, ____@____, ____@____, ____@____	
	____@____, ____@____, ____@____, ____@____, ____@____, ____@____	
	____@____, ____@____, ____@____, ____@____, ____@____, ____@____	
	____@____, ____@____, ____@____, ____@____, ____@____, ____@____	
	____@____, ____@____, ____@____, ____@____, ____@____, ____@____	

Mechanical Theme
Mob. > Corr. > Fun. Stability > NM Efficiency > Musc. Endurance > Hypertrophy > Heavy Power > Max Power > A.M.S.

Metabolic Theme
Met. Stim. > Aero. Elevation > Thresh. Development > Aero. Capacity > An. Expansion > Spec. Movements > Spec. Skills

Date	Warm Up		Cool Down		Movements/ Focus Area
	Exercise	*Duration*	*Exercise*	*Duration*	
___/___/___					

Activity	Rx (reps/dist. @ weight/time)	Rest
	____@____, ____@____, ____@____,	
	____@____, ____@____, ____@____	
	____@____, ____@____, ____@____,	
	____@____, ____@____, ____@____	
	____@____, ____@____, ____@____,	
	____@____, ____@____, ____@____	
	____@____, ____@____, ____@____,	
	____@____, ____@____, ____@____	
	____@____, ____@____, ____@____,	
	____@____, ____@____, ____@____	
	____@____, ____@____, ____@____,	
	____@____, ____@____, ____@____	
	____@____, ____@____, ____@____,	
	____@____, ____@____, ____@____	
	____@____, ____@____, ____@____,	
	____@____, ____@____, ____@____	
	____@____, ____@____, ____@____,	
	____@____, ____@____, ____@____	
	____@____, ____@____, ____@____,	
	____@____, ____@____, ____@____	
	____@____, ____@____, ____@____,	
	____@____, ____@____, ____@____	

Mechanical Theme
Mob. > Corr. > Fun. Stability > NM Efficiency > Musc. Endurance > Hypertrophy > Heavy Power > Max Power > A.M.S.

Metabolic Theme
Met. Stim. > Aero. Elevation > Thresh. Development > Aero. Capacity > An. Expansion > Spec. Movements > Spec. Skills

Date	Warm Up		Cool Down		Movements/ Focus Area
	Exercise	*Duration*	*Exercise*	*Duration*	
__/__/__					

Activity	Rx (reps/dist. @ weight/time)	Rest
	___@___ , ___@___ , ___@___ , ___@___ , ___@___ , ___@___	
	___@___ , ___@___ , ___@___ , ___@___ , ___@___ , ___@___	
	___@___ , ___@___ , ___@___ , ___@___ , ___@___ , ___@___	
	___@___ , ___@___ , ___@___ , ___@___ , ___@___ , ___@___	
	___@___ , ___@___ , ___@___ , ___@___ , ___@___ , ___@___	
	___@___ , ___@___ , ___@___ , ___@___ , ___@___ , ___@___	
	___@___ , ___@___ , ___@___ , ___@___ , ___@___ , ___@___	
	___@___ , ___@___ , ___@___ , ___@___ , ___@___ , ___@___	
	___@___ , ___@___ , ___@___ , ___@___ , ___@___ , ___@___	
	___@___ , ___@___ , ___@___ , ___@___ , ___@___ , ___@___	

Mechanical Theme
Mob. > Corr. > Fun. Stability > NM Efficiency > Musc. Endurance > Hypertrophy > Heavy Power > Max Power > A.M.S.

Metabolic Theme
Met. Stim. > Aero. Elevation > Thresh. Development > Aero. Capacity > An. Expansion > Spec. Movements > Spec. Skills

Date	Warm Up		Cool Down		Movements/ Focus Area
	Exercise	*Duration*	*Exercise*	*Duration*	
__ / __ / __					

Activity	Rx (reps/dist. @ weight/time)	Rest
	____ @ ____ , ____ @ ____ , ____ @ ____ ,	
	____ @ ____ , ____ @ ____ , ____ @ ____	
	____ @ ____ , ____ @ ____ , ____ @ ____ ,	
	____ @ ____ , ____ @ ____ , ____ @ ____	
	____ @ ____ , ____ @ ____ , ____ @ ____ ,	
	____ @ ____ , ____ @ ____ , ____ @ ____	
	____ @ ____ , ____ @ ____ , ____ @ ____ ,	
	____ @ ____ , ____ @ ____ , ____ @ ____	
	____ @ ____ , ____ @ ____ , ____ @ ____ ,	
	____ @ ____ , ____ @ ____ , ____ @ ____	
	____ @ ____ , ____ @ ____ , ____ @ ____ ,	
	____ @ ____ , ____ @ ____ , ____ @ ____	
	____ @ ____ , ____ @ ____ , ____ @ ____ ,	
	____ @ ____ , ____ @ ____ , ____ @ ____	
	____ @ ____ , ____ @ ____ , ____ @ ____ ,	
	____ @ ____ , ____ @ ____ , ____ @ ____	
	____ @ ____ , ____ @ ____ , ____ @ ____ ,	
	____ @ ____ , ____ @ ____ , ____ @ ____	
	____ @ ____ , ____ @ ____ , ____ @ ____ ,	
	____ @ ____ , ____ @ ____ , ____ @ ____	
	____ @ ____ , ____ @ ____ , ____ @ ____ ,	
	____ @ ____ , ____ @ ____ , ____ @ ____	

Mechanical Theme			
Mob. > Corr. > Fun. Stability > NM Efficiency > Musc. Endurance > Hypertrophy > Heavy Power > Max Power > A.M.S.			

Metabolic Theme			
Met. Stim. > Aero. Elevation > Thresh. Development > Aero. Capacity > An. Expansion > Spec. Movements > Spec. Skills			

Date	Warm Up		Cool Down		Movements/ Focus Area
	Exercise	*Duration*	*Exercise*	*Duration*	
___ / ___ / ___					

Activity	Rx (reps/dist. @ weight/time)	Rest
	____@____ , ____@____ , ____@____ , ____@____ , ____@____ , ____@____	
	____@____ , ____@____ , ____@____ , ____@____ , ____@____ , ____@____	
	____@____ , ____@____ , ____@____ , ____@____ , ____@____ , ____@____	
	____@____ , ____@____ , ____@____ , ____@____ , ____@____ , ____@____	
	____@____ , ____@____ , ____@____ , ____@____ , ____@____ , ____@____	
	____@____ , ____@____ , ____@____ , ____@____ , ____@____ , ____@____	
	____@____ , ____@____ , ____@____ , ____@____ , ____@____ , ____@____	
	____@____ , ____@____ , ____@____ , ____@____ , ____@____ , ____@____	
	____@____ , ____@____ , ____@____ , ____@____ , ____@____ , ____@____	
	____@____ , ____@____ , ____@____ , ____@____ , ____@____ , ____@____	
	____@____ , ____@____ , ____@____ , ____@____ , ____@____ , ____@____	

Mechanical Theme
Mob. > Corr. > Fun. Stability > NM Efficiency > Musc. Endurance > Hypertrophy > Heavy Power > Max Power > A.M.S.

Metabolic Theme
Met. Stim. > Aero. Elevation > Thresh. Development > Aero. Capacity > An. Expansion > Spec. Movements > Spec. Skills

Date	Warm Up		Cool Down		Movements/ Focus Area
	Exercise	*Duration*	*Exercise*	*Duration*	
___/___/___					

Activity	Rx (reps/dist. @ weight/time)	Rest
	____@____, ____@____, ____@____,	
	____@____, ____@____, ____@____	
	____@____, ____@____, ____@____,	
	____@____, ____@____, ____@____	
	____@____, ____@____, ____@____,	
	____@____, ____@____, ____@____	
	____@____, ____@____, ____@____,	
	____@____, ____@____, ____@____	
	____@____, ____@____, ____@____,	
	____@____, ____@____, ____@____	
	____@____, ____@____, ____@____,	
	____@____, ____@____, ____@____	
	____@____, ____@____, ____@____,	
	____@____, ____@____, ____@____	
	____@____, ____@____, ____@____,	
	____@____, ____@____, ____@____	
	____@____, ____@____, ____@____,	
	____@____, ____@____, ____@____	
	____@____, ____@____, ____@____,	
	____@____, ____@____, ____@____	

Mechanical Theme

Mob. > Corr. > Fun. Stability > NM Efficiency > Musc. Endurance > Hypertrophy > Heavy Power > Max Power > A.M.S.

Metabolic Theme
Met. Stim. > Aero. Elevation > Thresh. Development > Aero. Capacity > An. Expansion > Spec. Movements > Spec. Skills

Date	Warm Up		Cool Down		Movements/ Focus Area
	Exercise	*Duration*	*Exercise*	*Duration*	
___/___/___					

Activity	Rx (reps/dist. @ weight/time)	Rest
	___@___, ___@___, ___@___, ___@___, ___@___, ___@___	
	___@___, ___@___, ___@___, ___@___, ___@___, ___@___	
	___@___, ___@___, ___@___, ___@___, ___@___, ___@___	
	___@___, ___@___, ___@___, ___@___, ___@___, ___@___	
	___@___, ___@___, ___@___, ___@___, ___@___, ___@___	
	___@___, ___@___, ___@___, ___@___, ___@___, ___@___	
	___@___, ___@___, ___@___, ___@___, ___@___, ___@___	
	___@___, ___@___, ___@___, ___@___, ___@___, ___@___	
	___@___, ___@___, ___@___, ___@___, ___@___, ___@___	
	___@___, ___@___, ___@___, ___@___, ___@___, ___@___	

Mechanical Theme				
Mob. > Corr. > Fun. Stability > NM Efficiency > Musc. Endurance > Hypertrophy > Heavy Power > Max Power > A.M.S.				

Metabolic Theme				
Met. Stim. > Aero. Elevation > Thresh. Development > Aero. Capacity > An. Expansion > Spec. Movements > Spec. Skills				

Date	Warm Up		Cool Down		Movements/ Focus Area
	Exercise	*Duration*	*Exercise*	*Duration*	
___ / ___ / ___					

Activity	Rx (reps/dist. @ weight/time)	Rest
	____@____ , ____@____ , ____@____ ,	
	____@____ , ____@____ , ____@____	
	____@____ , ____@____ , ____@____ ,	
	____@____ , ____@____ , ____@____	
	____@____ , ____@____ , ____@____ ,	
	____@____ , ____@____ , ____@____	
	____@____ , ____@____ , ____@____ ,	
	____@____ , ____@____ , ____@____	
	____@____ , ____@____ , ____@____ ,	
	____@____ , ____@____ , ____@____	
	____@____ , ____@____ , ____@____ ,	
	____@____ , ____@____ , ____@____	
	____@____ , ____@____ , ____@____ ,	
	____@____ , ____@____ , ____@____	
	____@____ , ____@____ , ____@____ ,	
	____@____ , ____@____ , ____@____	
	____@____ , ____@____ , ____@____ ,	
	____@____ , ____@____ , ____@____	
	____@____ , ____@____ , ____@____ ,	
	____@____ , ____@____ , ____@____	
	____@____ , ____@____ , ____@____ ,	
	____@____ , ____@____ , ____@____	

Mechanical Theme
Mob. > Corr. > Fun. Stability > NM Efficiency > Musc. Endurance > Hypertrophy > Heavy Power > Max Power > A.M.S.

Metabolic Theme
Met. Stim. > Aero. Elevation > Thresh. Development > Aero. Capacity > An. Expansion > Spec. Movements > Spec. Skills

Date	Warm Up		Cool Down		Movements/ Focus Area
	Exercise	*Duration*	*Exercise*	*Duration*	
___/___/___					

Activity	Rx (reps/dist. @ weight/time)	Rest
	____@____, ____@____, ____@____, ____@____, ____@____, ____@____	
	____@____, ____@____, ____@____, ____@____, ____@____, ____@____	
	____@____, ____@____, ____@____, ____@____, ____@____, ____@____	
	____@____, ____@____, ____@____, ____@____, ____@____, ____@____	
	____@____, ____@____, ____@____, ____@____, ____@____, ____@____	
	____@____, ____@____, ____@____, ____@____, ____@____, ____@____	
	____@____, ____@____, ____@____, ____@____, ____@____, ____@____	
	____@____, ____@____, ____@____, ____@____, ____@____, ____@____	
	____@____, ____@____, ____@____, ____@____, ____@____, ____@____	
	____@____, ____@____, ____@____, ____@____, ____@____, ____@____	
	____@____, ____@____, ____@____, ____@____, ____@____, ____@____	

Mechanical Theme			
Mob. > Corr. > Fun. Stability > NM Efficiency > Musc. Endurance > Hypertrophy > Heavy Power > Max Power > A.M.S.			

Metabolic Theme			
Met. Stim. > Aero. Elevation > Thresh. Development > Aero. Capacity > An. Expansion > Spec. Movements > Spec. Skills			

Date	Warm Up		Cool Down		Movements/ Focus Area
	Exercise	*Duration*	*Exercise*	*Duration*	
___/___/___					

Activity	Rx (reps/dist. @ weight/time)	Rest
	___@___, ___@___, ___@___,	
	___@___, ___@___, ___@___	
	___@___, ___@___, ___@___,	
	___@___, ___@___, ___@___	
	___@___, ___@___, ___@___,	
	___@___, ___@___, ___@___	
	___@___, ___@___, ___@___,	
	___@___, ___@___, ___@___	
	___@___, ___@___, ___@___,	
	___@___, ___@___, ___@___	
	___@___, ___@___, ___@___,	
	___@___, ___@___, ___@___	
	___@___, ___@___, ___@___,	
	___@___, ___@___, ___@___	
	___@___, ___@___, ___@___,	
	___@___, ___@___, ___@___	
	___@___, ___@___, ___@___,	
	___@___, ___@___, ___@___	
	___@___, ___@___, ___@___,	
	___@___, ___@___, ___@___	
	___@___, ___@___, ___@___,	
	___@___, ___@___, ___@___	

Mechanical Theme					
Mob. > Corr. > Fun. Stability > NM Efficiency > Musc. Endurance > Hypertrophy > Heavy Power > Max Power > A.M.S.					

Metabolic Theme			
Met. Stim. > Aero. Elevation > Thresh. Development > Aero. Capacity > An. Expansion > Spec. Movements > Spec. Skills			

Date	Warm Up		Cool Down		Movements/ Focus Area
	Exercise	*Duration*	*Exercise*	*Duration*	
___/___/___					

Activity	Rx (reps/dist. @ weight/time)	Rest
	____@____ , ____@____ , ____@____ ,	
	____@____ , ____@____ , ____@____	
	____@____ , ____@____ , ____@____ ,	
	____@____ , ____@____ , ____@____	
	____@____ , ____@____ , ____@____ ,	
	____@____ , ____@____ , ____@____	
	____@____ , ____@____ , ____@____ ,	
	____@____ , ____@____ , ____@____	
	____@____ , ____@____ , ____@____ ,	
	____@____ , ____@____ , ____@____	
	____@____ , ____@____ , ____@____ ,	
	____@____ , ____@____ , ____@____	
	____@____ , ____@____ , ____@____ ,	
	____@____ , ____@____ , ____@____	
	____@____ , ____@____ , ____@____ ,	
	____@____ , ____@____ , ____@____	
	____@____ , ____@____ , ____@____ ,	
	____@____ , ____@____ , ____@____	
	____@____ , ____@____ , ____@____ ,	
	____@____ , ____@____ , ____@____	

Mechanical Theme
Mob. > Corr. > Fun. Stability > NM Efficiency > Musc. Endurance > Hypertrophy > Heavy Power > Max Power > A.M.S.

Metabolic Theme
Met. Stim. > Aero. Elevation > Thresh. Development > Aero. Capacity > An. Expansion > Spec. Movements > Spec. Skills

Date	Warm Up		Cool Down		Movements/ Focus Area
	Exercise	*Duration*	*Exercise*	*Duration*	
___/___/___					

Activity	Rx (reps/dist. @ weight/time)	Rest
	___@___, ___@___, ___@___,	
	___@___, ___@___, ___@___	
	___@___, ___@___, ___@___,	
	___@___, ___@___, ___@___	
	___@___, ___@___, ___@___,	
	___@___, ___@___, ___@___	
	___@___, ___@___, ___@___,	
	___@___, ___@___, ___@___	
	___@___, ___@___, ___@___,	
	___@___, ___@___, ___@___	
	___@___, ___@___, ___@___,	
	___@___, ___@___, ___@___	
	___@___, ___@___, ___@___,	
	___@___, ___@___, ___@___	
	___@___, ___@___, ___@___,	
	___@___, ___@___, ___@___	
	___@___, ___@___, ___@___,	
	___@___, ___@___, ___@___	
	___@___, ___@___, ___@___,	
	___@___, ___@___, ___@___	
	___@___, ___@___, ___@___,	
	___@___, ___@___, ___@___	

Mechanical Theme
Mob. > Corr. > Fun. Stability > NM Efficiency > Musc. Endurance > Hypertrophy > Heavy Power > Max Power > A.M.S.

Metabolic Theme
Met. Stim. > Aero. Elevation > Thresh. Development > Aero. Capacity > An. Expansion > Spec. Movements > Spec. Skills

Date	Warm Up		Cool Down		Movements/ Focus Area
	Exercise	*Duration*	*Exercise*	*Duration*	
__ / __ / __					

Activity	Rx (reps/dist. @ weight/time)	Rest
	___@___, ___@___, ___@___, ___@___, ___@___, ___@___	
	___@___, ___@___, ___@___, ___@___, ___@___, ___@___	
	___@___, ___@___, ___@___, ___@___, ___@___, ___@___	
	___@___, ___@___, ___@___, ___@___, ___@___, ___@___	
	___@___, ___@___, ___@___, ___@___, ___@___, ___@___	
	___@___, ___@___, ___@___, ___@___, ___@___, ___@___	
	___@___, ___@___, ___@___, ___@___, ___@___, ___@___	
	___@___, ___@___, ___@___, ___@___, ___@___, ___@___	
	___@___, ___@___, ___@___, ___@___, ___@___, ___@___	
	___@___, ___@___, ___@___, ___@___, ___@___, ___@___	

Mechanical Theme
Mob. > Corr. > Fun. Stability > NM Efficiency > Musc. Endurance > Hypertrophy > Heavy Power > Max Power > A.M.S.

Metabolic Theme
Met. Stim. > Aero. Elevation > Thresh. Development > Aero. Capacity > An. Expansion > Spec. Movements > Spec. Skills

Date	Warm Up		Cool Down		Movements/ Focus Area
	Exercise	*Duration*	*Exercise*	*Duration*	
__ / __ / __					

Activity	Rx (reps/dist. @ weight/time)	Rest
	____@____, ____@____, ____@____,	
	____@____, ____@____, ____@____	
	____@____, ____@____, ____@____,	
	____@____, ____@____, ____@____	
	____@____, ____@____, ____@____,	
	____@____, ____@____, ____@____	
	____@____, ____@____, ____@____,	
	____@____, ____@____, ____@____	
	____@____, ____@____, ____@____,	
	____@____, ____@____, ____@____	
	____@____, ____@____, ____@____,	
	____@____, ____@____, ____@____	
	____@____, ____@____, ____@____,	
	____@____, ____@____, ____@____	
	____@____, ____@____, ____@____,	
	____@____, ____@____, ____@____	
	____@____, ____@____, ____@____,	
	____@____, ____@____, ____@____	
	____@____, ____@____, ____@____,	
	____@____, ____@____, ____@____	

Mechanical Theme
Mob. > Corr. > Fun. Stability > NM Efficiency > Musc. Endurance > Hypertrophy > Heavy Power > Max Power > A.M.S.

Metabolic Theme
Met. Stim. > Aero. Elevation > Thresh. Development > Aero. Capacity > An. Expansion > Spec. Movements > Spec. Skills

Date	Warm Up		Cool Down		Movements/ Focus Area
	Exercise	*Duration*	*Exercise*	*Duration*	
___/___/___					

Activity	**Rx** (reps/dist. @ weight/time)	Rest
	____@____, ____@____, ____@____, ____@____, ____@____, ____@____	
	____@____, ____@____, ____@____, ____@____, ____@____, ____@____	
	____@____, ____@____, ____@____, ____@____, ____@____, ____@____	
	____@____, ____@____, ____@____, ____@____, ____@____, ____@____	
	____@____, ____@____, ____@____, ____@____, ____@____, ____@____	
	____@____, ____@____, ____@____, ____@____, ____@____, ____@____	
	____@____, ____@____, ____@____, ____@____, ____@____, ____@____	
	____@____, ____@____, ____@____, ____@____, ____@____, ____@____	
	____@____, ____@____, ____@____, ____@____, ____@____, ____@____	
	____@____, ____@____, ____@____, ____@____, ____@____, ____@____	

Mechanical Theme				
Mob. > Corr. > Fun. Stability > NM Efficiency > Musc. Endurance > Hypertrophy > Heavy Power > Max Power > A.M.S.				
Metabolic Theme				
Met. Stim. > Aero. Elevation > Thresh. Development > Aero. Capacity > An. Expansion > Spec. Movements > Spec. Skills				

Date	Warm Up		Cool Down		Movements/ Focus Area
	Exercise	_Duration_	_Exercise_	_Duration_	
___/___/___					

Activity	Rx (reps/dist. @ weight/time)	Rest
	____@____, ____@____, ____@____,	
	____@____, ____@____, ____@____	
	____@____, ____@____, ____@____,	
	____@____, ____@____, ____@____	
	____@____, ____@____, ____@____,	
	____@____, ____@____, ____@____	
	____@____, ____@____, ____@____,	
	____@____, ____@____, ____@____	
	____@____, ____@____, ____@____,	
	____@____, ____@____, ____@____	
	____@____, ____@____, ____@____,	
	____@____, ____@____, ____@____	
	____@____, ____@____, ____@____,	
	____@____, ____@____, ____@____	
	____@____, ____@____, ____@____,	
	____@____, ____@____, ____@____	
	____@____, ____@____, ____@____,	
	____@____, ____@____, ____@____	
	____@____, ____@____, ____@____,	
	____@____, ____@____, ____@____	

Mechanical Theme
Mob. > Corr. > Fun. Stability > NM Efficiency > Musc. Endurance > Hypertrophy > Heavy Power > Max Power > A.M.S.

Metabolic Theme
Met. Stim. > Aero. Elevation > Thresh. Development > Aero. Capacity > An. Expansion > Spec. Movements > Spec. Skills

Date	Warm Up		Cool Down		Movements/ Focus Area
	Exercise	*Duration*	*Exercise*	*Duration*	
___ / ___ / ___					

Activity	Rx (reps/dist. @ weight/time)	Rest
	____@____, ____@____, ____@____, ____@____, ____@____, ____@____	
	____@____, ____@____, ____@____, ____@____, ____@____, ____@____	
	____@____, ____@____, ____@____, ____@____, ____@____, ____@____	
	____@____, ____@____, ____@____, ____@____, ____@____, ____@____	
	____@____, ____@____, ____@____, ____@____, ____@____, ____@____	
	____@____, ____@____, ____@____, ____@____, ____@____, ____@____	
	____@____, ____@____, ____@____, ____@____, ____@____, ____@____	
	____@____, ____@____, ____@____, ____@____, ____@____, ____@____	
	____@____, ____@____, ____@____, ____@____, ____@____, ____@____	
	____@____, ____@____, ____@____, ____@____, ____@____, ____@____	

Mechanical Theme
Mob. > Corr. > Fun. Stability > NM Efficiency > Musc. Endurance > Hypertrophy > Heavy Power > Max Power > A.M.S.

Metabolic Theme
Met. Stim. > Aero. Elevation > Thresh. Development > Aero. Capacity > An. Expansion > Spec. Movements > Spec. Skills

Date	Warm Up		Cool Down		Movements/ Focus Area
	Exercise	*Duration*	*Exercise*	*Duration*	
___ / ___ / ___					

Activity	Rx (reps/dist. @ weight/time)			Rest
	___ @ ___ ,	___ @ ___ ,	___ @ ___ ,	
	___ @ ___ ,	___ @ ___ ,	___ @ ___	
	___ @ ___ ,	___ @ ___ ,	___ @ ___ ,	
	___ @ ___ ,	___ @ ___ ,	___ @ ___	
	___ @ ___ ,	___ @ ___ ,	___ @ ___ ,	
	___ @ ___ ,	___ @ ___ ,	___ @ ___	
	___ @ ___ ,	___ @ ___ ,	___ @ ___ ,	
	___ @ ___ ,	___ @ ___ ,	___ @ ___	
	___ @ ___ ,	___ @ ___ ,	___ @ ___ ,	
	___ @ ___ ,	___ @ ___ ,	___ @ ___	
	___ @ ___ ,	___ @ ___ ,	___ @ ___ ,	
	___ @ ___ ,	___ @ ___ ,	___ @ ___	
	___ @ ___ ,	___ @ ___ ,	___ @ ___ ,	
	___ @ ___ ,	___ @ ___ ,	___ @ ___	
	___ @ ___ ,	___ @ ___ ,	___ @ ___ ,	
	___ @ ___ ,	___ @ ___ ,	___ @ ___	
	___ @ ___ ,	___ @ ___ ,	___ @ ___ ,	
	___ @ ___ ,	___ @ ___ ,	___ @ ___	
	___ @ ___ ,	___ @ ___ ,	___ @ ___ ,	
	___ @ ___ ,	___ @ ___ ,	___ @ ___	

Mechanical Theme
Mob. > Corr. > Fun. Stability > NM Efficiency > Musc. Endurance > Hypertrophy > Heavy Power > Max Power > A.M.S.

Metabolic Theme
Met. Stim. > Aero. Elevation > Thresh. Development > Aero. Capacity > An. Expansion > Spec. Movements > Spec. Skills

Date	Warm Up		Cool Down		Movements/ Focus Area
	Exercise	*Duration*	*Exercise*	*Duration*	
__/__/__					

Activity	**Rx** (reps/dist. @ weight/time)	Rest
	___@___, ___@___, ___@___, ___@___, ___@___, ___@___	
	___@___, ___@___, ___@___, ___@___, ___@___, ___@___	
	___@___, ___@___, ___@___, ___@___, ___@___, ___@___	
	___@___, ___@___, ___@___, ___@___, ___@___, ___@___	
	___@___, ___@___, ___@___, ___@___, ___@___, ___@___	
	___@___, ___@___, ___@___, ___@___, ___@___, ___@___	
	___@___, ___@___, ___@___, ___@___, ___@___, ___@___	
	___@___, ___@___, ___@___, ___@___, ___@___, ___@___	
	___@___, ___@___, ___@___, ___@___, ___@___, ___@___	
	___@___, ___@___, ___@___, ___@___, ___@___, ___@___	

Mechanical Theme
Mob. > Corr. > Fun. Stability > NM Efficiency > Musc. Endurance > Hypertrophy > Heavy Power > Max Power > A.M.S.

Metabolic Theme
Met. Stim. > Aero. Elevation > Thresh. Development > Aero. Capacity > An. Expansion > Spec. Movements > Spec. Skills

Date	Warm Up		Cool Down		Movements/ Focus Area
	Exercise	*Duration*	*Exercise*	*Duration*	
___/___/___					

Activity	Rx (reps/dist. @ weight/time)	Rest
	___@____, ____@____, ____@____,	
	___@____, ____@____, ____@____	
	___@____, ____@____, ____@____,	
	___@____, ____@____, ____@____	
	___@____, ____@____, ____@____,	
	___@____, ____@____, ____@____	
	___@____, ____@____, ____@____,	
	___@____, ____@____, ____@____	
	___@____, ____@____, ____@____,	
	___@____, ____@____, ____@____	
	___@____, ____@____, ____@____,	
	___@____, ____@____, ____@____	
	___@____, ____@____, ____@____,	
	___@____, ____@____, ____@____	
	___@____, ____@____, ____@____,	
	___@____, ____@____, ____@____	
	___@____, ____@____, ____@____,	
	___@____, ____@____, ____@____	
	___@____, ____@____, ____@____,	
	___@____, ____@____, ____@____	

Mechanical Theme
Mob. > Corr. > Fun. Stability > NM Efficiency > Musc. Endurance > Hypertrophy > Heavy Power > Max Power > A.M.S.

Metabolic Theme
Met. Stim. > Aero. Elevation > Thresh. Development > Aero. Capacity > An. Expansion > Spec. Movements > Spec. Skills

Date	Warm Up		Cool Down		Movements/ Focus Area
	Exercise	*Duration*	*Exercise*	*Duration*	
___/___/___					

Activity	Rx (reps/dist. @ weight/time)	Rest
	___@___, ___@___, ___@___, ___@___, ___@___, ___@___	
	___@___, ___@___, ___@___, ___@___, ___@___, ___@___	
	___@___, ___@___, ___@___, ___@___, ___@___, ___@___	
	___@___, ___@___, ___@___, ___@___, ___@___, ___@___	
	___@___, ___@___, ___@___, ___@___, ___@___, ___@___	
	___@___, ___@___, ___@___, ___@___, ___@___, ___@___	
	___@___, ___@___, ___@___, ___@___, ___@___, ___@___	
	___@___, ___@___, ___@___, ___@___, ___@___, ___@___	
	___@___, ___@___, ___@___, ___@___, ___@___, ___@___	
	___@___, ___@___, ___@___, ___@___, ___@___, ___@___	

Client PROgress stamp 1

Date___/___/___

Resting HR_____   Max HR_____   Blood Pressure____/____   Cholesterol_____

Measurements

Weight_____Lbs / kg   Waist_____in /cm

Neck_____in / cm   Hip_____in /cm

Calf_____in / cm   Thigh_____in / cm

Chest_____in / cm   Upper Arms_____in / cm

BMI_____   Body Composition_____%

1RM

Back Squat_____Lbs / kg   Deadlift_____Lbs / kg

Bench Press_____Lbs / kg   Incline Bench Press_____Lbs / kg

Bent Over Row_____Lbs / kg   Pull up_____Reps

Cardiovascular

10m Acceleration_____sec   40m Sprint_____sec

T-Test_____sec   300m Shuttle Run_____sec

1 mile Run_____(min:sec)   2 mile Run_____(min:sec)

5k Run_____(min:sec)   2,000m Row_____(min:sec)

100 Flights of Staris_____(min:sec)

Additional Notes:

Client PROgress stamp 2

Date___/___/___

Resting HR_____   Max HR_____   Blood Pressure____/____   Cholesterol_____

Measurements

Weight_____Lbs / kg   Waist_____in /cm

Neck_____in / cm   Hip_____in /cm

Calf_____in / cm   Thigh_____in / cm

Chest_____in / cm   Upper Arms_____in / cm

BMI_____   Body Composition_____%

1RM

Back Squat_____Lbs / kg   Deadlift_____Lbs / kg

Bench Press_____Lbs / kg   Incline Bench Press_____Lbs / kg

Bent Over Row_____Lbs / kg   Pull up_____Reps

Cardiovascular

10m Acceleration_____sec   40m Sprint_____sec

T-Test_____sec   300m Shuttle Run_____sec

1 mile Run_____(min:sec)   2 mile Run_____(min:sec)

5k Run_____(min:sec)   2,000m Row_____(min:sec)

100 Flights of Staris_____(min:sec)

Additional Notes:

Client PROgress stamp 3

Date___/___/___

Resting HR_____   Max HR_____   Blood Pressure____/____   Cholesterol_____

Measurements

Weight_____Lbs / kg   Waist_____in /cm

Neck_____in / cm   Hip_____in /cm

Calf_____in / cm   Thigh_____in / cm

Chest_____in / cm   Upper Arms_____in / cm

BMI_____   Body Composition_____%

1RM

Back Squat_____Lbs / kg   Deadlift_____Lbs / kg

Bench Press_____Lbs / kg   Incline Bench Press_____Lbs / kg

Bent Over Row_____Lbs / kg   Pull up_____Reps

Cardiovascular

10m Acceleration_____sec   40m Sprint_____sec

T-Test_____sec   300m Shuttle Run_____sec

1 mile Run_____(min:sec)   2 mile Run_____(min:sec)

5k Run_____(min:sec)   2,000m Row_____(min:sec)

100 Flights of Staris_____(min:sec)

Additional Notes:

PR (Personal Records)

Date	Activity	PR (Personal Record)	Notes

Notes

www.ingramcontent.com/pod-product-compliance
Lightning Source LLC
Chambersburg PA
CBHW080420290526
45791CB00008BA/2354